D1454083

A PINCH OF THYME:
Easy Lessons For
a Leaner Life

by

Robyn Webb

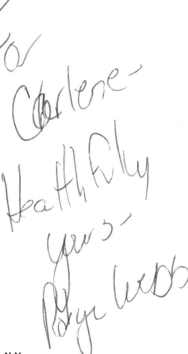

For
Carlene—
Healthfuly
yours,
Robyn Webb

KENDALL/HUNT PUBLISHING COMPANY
4050 Westmark Drive   Dubuque, Iowa 52002

ISBN 0-8403-9384-9

Printed in the United States of America

10   9   8   7   6   5   4   3   2   1

Table of Contents

Table of Contents

FOREWORD

I love Robyn Webb...and the recipes that come out of her kitchen.

I've known her for years—long before she opened her hugely successful cooking school, *A Pinch of Thyme*, in Old Town Alexandria, Virginia, and long before the idea of writing a low-fat, low-sugar cookbook was even a gleam in her eyes.

And yet Robyn continues to surprise me! For instance, Robyn can take ordinary ingredients and turn them into something extraordinary. She constantly shows kitchen creativity that most of us can only aspire to. Yet day after day she finds the way to meld healthy and delicious into the same mouthful.

It's remarkable how her recipes reflect who she is. Her sense of fun is evident as she combines unusual flavors, textures, aromas and foods to make an exceptional dish. Her sense of adventure peeks through when she counterpoints the everyday with the exotic. Her sense of order shows as she clearly takes a novice through a step-by-step approach to food preparation. Her self-confidence in tackling such a project in the first place—well, what more can I say!

But what I admire most about Robyn Webb and the wonderful foods she creates for our pleasure is that no matter how delicious they are, no matter how beautiful to look at, they are low in fat and low in sugar. And that means *healthy.*

As a nutritionist, I heartily recommend the healthy cooking style Robyn teaches in *A Pinch of Thyme.* As a friend of the author, who savored many of the recipes before they saw print, I urge you to try them for yourself. You'll eat well and feel better.

Bon appetit!

Sara Blumenthal, L.N., Washington, D.C.
Licensed Nutritionist in Private Practice

NUTRITIONAL NOTE FOR ALL RECIPIES

Nutritional analysis of each recipe is available by calling 1-800-374-1471, or writing to: Robyn Webb Associates; 325 N. West Street; Alexandria, VA 22314. The analysis is not included at this time, primarily because we want you to enjoy the food rather than simply eating by the *numbers*. Rest assured, all recipes are appropriate for anyone watching fat intake, and we are always happy to provide specific nutritional information.

Ready? Begin your lessons for a leaner life.

DEDICATION

This book is lovingly dedicated

To my mother, Ruth, who allowed me to play with pots and pans as a baby and who continues to stand by me everyday;

To my husband, Allan, who puts up with my never being home because I am out cooking for everyone else but him.

I love you both!

ACKNOWLEDGMENTS

Many heartfelt thanks go to the people behind the scenes of this book, many of whom have supported me throughout the years.

To the staff at Kendall/Hunt Publishing Company, particularly David Metcalf. His expertise in the area of publishing helped to coordinate the process of this book—professionally and with ease.

To my editor, contributing writer, and friend, Daniel Herlong, for his partnership and his belief that this project is needed and wanted.

To my publicist, Amy Cubbard Katz, for her undying commitment to the growth of my business and her extraordinary talent and ability to transform words into gold.

To outstanding graphic designers, Amy Howell and Sandy Hettler, for their sense of beauty and creativity in designs for our many projects over the years.

To Janet Zalman, my employer before I began my own business and one of the top and best nutritionists in Washington, D.C., for the chance to develop my potential as a teacher and an opportunity to *spread my wings.*

To Sara Blumenthal, for not only writing an eloquent forward for this book, but for her long-time friendship and her continued belief in me. If there were more nutritionists like Sara, there would be less disease and sickness in this country.

To Arnold Sanow, *Mr. Marketing*, my management consultant. For without him, neither my business nor this book would exist.

To Laura Griffin Farrell, my first office assistant, for her encouragement to write and for her presence when it all began.

To Kelly Johnson, Loretta Colom, and Yvonne Chanatry, whose support, great ideas, and staying-power through challenging times will never be forgotten.

Finally and most importantly, to my clients whose lives I have been able to touch and who have reaped benefit from my work, I am very proud and honored to know each of you.

A PERSONAL NOTE FROM ROBYN

After much begging, pleading, and cajoling from my clients, I am finally writing my book! Part of my initial hesitation was a concern that I did not want a book that would collect dust on a shelf or adorn a coffee table unopened. After years of teaching, my clients have reassured me, they do use my recipes in everyday cooking, and they find them easy to follow, utilizing common ingredients, and consistently appealing and delicious! After class participation, many clients tell me that they feel inspired—that the manner in which I teach enables even the clumsiest neophyte to become a stove top Stravinsky! I have realized that I do want to present the same streamlined, practical information in written words.

This personal note is to explain the format and to present a short *user* guide, which may facilitate your enjoyment and enhance your recognition of the many benefits this book has to offer.

The book is divided into two parts. The first part shares with you my struggle with weight and health, and how I was able to begin on a road of permanent weight and health management. It discusses ways we can motivate ourselves to become and stay healthy. It touches on everyday situations that are difficult and strategies to overcome them.

The second part includes resources for wonderful foods, cooking charts, and the procedure for stocking a pantry correctly. It also offers some of my favorite recipes. My next book will include more. I want to discover what my readers may prefer next time.

Let me tell you what is not included in this book and why. I don't go deeply into the science of nutrition or explanations of what you should eat everyday. For one thing, there are many people who *know* a lot about nutrition but don't do anything specific about improving their health. They are missing the skills that make the difference between just *knowing* and actually *doing*. My intention is that this book will give some practical tools to alleviate this situation and to help you get started. I have purposely eliminated strict guidelines on what *should* be eaten everyday because everyone is different. Nutrition is a very personal and specific science. The same rules do not apply to everyone. Sure, there are some generally good guidelines everyone can follow, but let us be careful to treat everyone as an individual with precise needs.

You can get more out of this book, if you utilize the short *user's* guide that I have established for your convenience.

1. GIVE YOURSELF CREDIT - YOU bought this book. I acknowledge that action as a commitment to improve your health (at least I know that you are curious enough to buy it!). When you start to feel better and to create meals that take a minimal amount of time and effort to prepare, give yourself a big pat on the back! If you want to *pay* me back, write or call me and let me know how you are doing.

2. FEEL FREE TO EXPERIMENT AND HAVE FUN - Did I say fun, experiment? Two words many people never use to describe cooking! My recipes are designed so that you can vary ingredients, add more or less of something, and not pay too much attention to the painstaking techniques of perfect chopping, slicing, and dicing! I want you to have fun and feel comfortable just being in the kitchen. We'll worry about the exact diameter-cut of your carrot later on.

3. ASK FOR SUPPORT - Even if you have never met me, please call or write to me and ask lots of questions! If you are having any trouble with the recipes, can't locate an ingredient, want more nutritional information or just want to chat, don't be a stranger. Tell me what you want included in my next book too!

Let's begin the adventure! Turn the page and start!

Healthfully yours,

Robyn

ABOUT THE AUTHOR

Robyn Webb, M.S., is President of Robyn Webb Associates, a one-stop source for all your nutritional needs. Her expertise in the field of nutrition and cooking has been featured in articles by Woman's Day Magazine, Cosmopolitan Magazine, Associated Press, Virginia Business Magazine, Alexandria Gazette, Washingtonian Magazine, The Washington Business Journal, USA Today, and The Washington Post. Robyn Webb has appeared nationally on CBS news with Dan Rather and on ESPN with Denise Austin, fitness expert, Broadcast House Live on WUSA TV Channel 9, WRC-TV, Channel 4 with Susan Kidd and Lea Thompson's five week FIGHTING FAT series, WJLA Channel 7 News and Working Woman.

Robyn Webb regularly lectures to Washington area companies and organizations and is a regular lecturer for Fresh Fields stores. She has also developed an educational audiocassette *40 Ways to Cut Fat*, designed to teach people how to lower the fat content of food without sacrificing taste.

Robyn Webb received her Master of Science degree in nutrition from Florida State University and has been successfully engaged in the field of nutrition for over ten years. She lives in Old Town, Alexandria, Virginia with her husband Allan.

PART I

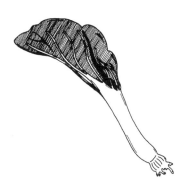

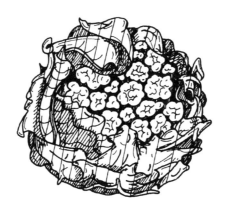

CHAPTER 1

My Turn

I grew up in a household that specialized in an over-abundance of delicious food! Although good quality food was emphasized, I always had a weight problem. After about the fifth attempt to lose weight with weird and crazy diets, I knew I had to find a better way. I was tired of yo-yoing weight and dress sizes and never feeling really well. Then I realized I had to make a commitment for the rest of my life in order to turn things around and live the life I wanted. My food philosophy has evolved and now I see nutrition as something that you can't just *do*, but rather, you must really *live it as a lifestyle!*

Although the last time I tried to take weight off, it took me longer than it had in the past, I was able to keep off the weight I eventually lost. With my weight reduced and my eating habits improved, I found that my whole outlook on life changed. I realized that nutrition was not something you could put on a *back burner* as a "could've, should've, would've" affair. It needed to be relegated to the *forefront* of life. When you eat well and exercise, your whole life becomes more positively oriented. I also realized that everything I wanted out of life could be accomplished if I had my health!

Watching my health is the most important, yet the hardest, thing I ever do. I manage to do everything else: I run a company; I deal with hundreds of people every week; and I do things that, normally, people would be afraid to attempt. But I continually struggle with putting my health into the center of it all—with making health the most important element of my life.

Filling the gap between "Knowing" and "Doing"

I really believe that people can't just pick up a nutrition book and say to themselves, "OK, now I'm going to start this and I'm going to be perfect." Understanding the value of nutrition is an evolving process. During my lectures I tell people that if they take one piece of advice and use it consistently over the course of a year and then, the next year remember something else that I said and use it for a year, pretty soon they will have an accumulation of all kinds of tips and hints that will make a difference. I have seen too many people the day after New Year's day, who say, "I'm going to join the health club," or "I'm going to hit the tread mill," "eat right and be healthy," and many other positive affirmations only to have it all end in three weeks. I think people today are smarter because the type of people I have been seeing in my lectures are more sophisticated than they used to be. But, it's interesting to note that with as much knowledge as we are gaining, with all the resources available—more nutritionists, health clubs, personal trainers, etc.—research continues to show that people are not eating wisely. The exercise craze seems to have hit a very visible minority, but the majority of people in this country still are not exercising. People seem to think reading a book will improve their health without putting the principles into action. They simply become confused by the myriad of information, some of it conflicting, and then they tend to do nothing.

Apple cider vinegar helps you lose weight. Eat lemons. Don't eat lemons. Exercise before you go to bed. Exercise when you wake up. Only eat eggs with grapefruit. Only eat fruit in the morning. Don't eat fruit in the morning. Trying to follow all that advice would drive anybody nuts. So people rationalize that when the experts get it all together and prove beyond a shadow of a doubt which process will improve health and to what degree, then they will indulge in the proper exercise and eat correctly. If people can figure out what works for them and stick with it, then that's good for them, but if things aren't going very well, maybe some evaluation of what they are doing is in order. I find that when people can be committed to concentrate on a few basics, they do much better.

If you are not yet ready to seriously embark on something that may take time and commitment, don't do anything crazy and stupid or go hog wild only to have good intentions backfire. Training people to recognize there is something at stake in their health is a very difficult thing to do. Ask yourself the question, why? Why do you want to lose weight? Without the answer to this question you really can't go anywhere. *I should, I want, somebody else did, somebody else thinks I should*, is not sufficient justification to do anything. The commitment to losing weight must be so important personally, that a person will do whatever it takes to accomplish this goal. This kind of personal, internal, positive motivation is mandatory. Sporadic, positive activity motivated by temporary pain and personal dissatisfaction can't last and sets up the yo-yo effect.

The biggest challenge to me in my nutritional practice is to teach people about internal motivation and commitment. The challenge exists because I am still learning what motivates me. My success is born out of reaching a point where I recognized that the quality of my life was not going in the direction that I had hoped for and then realizing that I had to do something about it. I can't put my finger on why I was successful, but I know that for the first time I was open to the possibility that maybe by making a lifetime change, I could turn myself around. I was skeptical as to whether or not I could make such a change, but I worked very, very hard accepting the challenge, and I hung in there. That's the best answer I have as to what it takes to be successful.

I have learned that persistence is the key to accomplishment. If people can use the successful areas of their lives as their model, possibly they can change those areas they wish to improve. Ask yourself, why am I successful in business, relationships, or sports? Maybe it's because I'm organized, write everything down, or can see the results. Whatever it is, can I use those methods in managing my health? I have very successful clients—entrepreneurs, presidents, and CEOs—highly intelligent people, who can't get their health and eating habits under control. In helping them, I always ask them to name seven things they consider responsible for their success in business. We then explore using those same things to manage their health. Using something that is familiar in one aspect of life can be carried over into other areas.

Making Friends with Food

Many people think that food is a separate part of their lives, but it's all the same one life we're living! I had one client who said, "Food is no different from anything else in my life, and the way that I keep my checkbook, make my bed, or brush my teeth is the way that I take care of my food. When my food is not working, my checkbook and bed are sloppy and I fight with my husband." I have come to the conclusion that it is absolutely holistic. Food has to work for life to be happy and healthy and there is no separating the two. The normal approach to a weight problem is to divorce oneself from eating and develop an anxiety toward food when the best approach is just the opposite. Food must be your friend and you must eat well (properly prepared, healthy foods) to lose weight.

So many diets say *don't do this, don't do that, don't, don't, don't!* Sure! There are some dont's, but more importantly, what is it that we can *do*?

How do you make friends with food so you can eat and lose weight? It's important to understand that food, cooking, and interest in food are not the enemies. Some people tell me they are going on a diet and so they're going to throw away all their cooking magazines! I say, "You don't have to do that; you don't have to do anything like that." If your interest in food is interfering with getting the results you desire, you may have to look into modifying certain behavior patterns surrounding food, but don't stop cooking or lose your interest in eating. My way has been to make food so important in my life that I developed a cooking school and I'm always talking and reading about food. There is nothing wrong with an interest in food, it just has to be channeled in such a way that it supports the desired end results. For me, if suddenly I took up an interest in cooking fabulous chocolate deserts, that just wouldn't fit into my program. I would have to get rid of it. At the same time, reading about a new herb, spice, or technique of preparing or cooking that supports my goals will help me enjoy my food. I've just seen so many people try to deny their interest in food until they are so overwhelmed that they just have to eat whatever is closest at hand (usually junk food). Interest in food is what can help you discover how to enjoy eating while losing those extra pounds. Practicing good nutrition is like being in a black hole; there are no limits, no end in sight. It doesn't stop when our cholesterol or our weight drops, or when we start to feel better about ourselves. It keeps on going and going and never, never ends! To quote the late, great British Prime Minister Winston Churchill: "Never, never, never give up!"

Can you benefit from better nutrition in your life? The answer is YES! I believe that nutrition is at the root of all life. You need to ask yourself some questions to determine how it can benefit you specifically. How do you feel? How much are you spending on medical bills? How many colds and sore throats have you had recently? Many people who are not overweight but just eke through their days don't really think about nutrition. They don't realize that they may have some problems down the road if they are eating poorly. Is there anything in your life that you feel you don't have enough energy for or any special accomplishment that eludes you? It's possible that some of the foods that you are eating are causing a problem. The trick is to relate nutrition to something that is really important to you. There are still people who don't believe nutrition makes a difference. But if you are eating well and exercising regularly, you will see every aspect of your life improve. I've seen enough success stories over the past ten years to guarantee that this is true!

Where Do You Start?

Probably the most beneficial, basic area—and the easiest to understand—is FAT. This area provides some of the most conclusive research available today. Fat is linked directly to obesity, high cholesterol, heart disease, sluggishness, and fatigue. Some people say, "OK, I'll just eat fat-free foods." This can be an improvement, but good health is so much more than that. It requires a holistic approach that also includes: stopping smoking, reducing stress, and eating good, wholesome food.

People need to start with eliminating the obvious sources of fat in their diet. Take a hard look at your cooking methods, i.e. deep fat-frying and stir frying with too much of the wrong kinds of oils. Instead, cook oil-free as much as possible and eliminate all the junk food from your diet; that will go a long way toward improving your fat intake. Then eliminate the butter, salad dressing, and high-fat dairy products. How many people go to a party and eat just one of those little cheese squares that contain, on the average, nine grams of fat? Ten, maybe? Have you lost count?

As a first step, try keeping a food diary for just a week. This will help you learn where fat is hidden in your diet; most people are very surprised and a bit humbled by this exercise! The recommendations from the American Heart Association are that we reduce our fat intake to 30% of our total calories, but I believe, to make a serious impact on health in our daily lives, that for most folks an intake of 20% is much better. I don't imply that anyone should try to achieve 20% immediately, but it can be done gradually. I have found that over time, as fat is reduced in the diet, the craving for the taste of fat diminishes. So if you are now consuming 60% of your calories as fat, cut it to 40% then 30% then shoot for the lowest amount that you can feel comfortable with. It's not just changing over to *fat-free* products (most of which have a great deal of sugar) and reading—often misleading—labels for fat content that will make a difference. It's changing your thinking to reflect a new understanding of how fat affects your life.

Our lives are very fast paced, and convenience foods are the easiest way to obtain sustenance. Unfortunately, these are high in fat. As human beings we are accustomed to the taste of fat, and it tastes particularly good to us. We crave it. The texture of fat feels comforting and many use it to reduce the feeling of stress and to ward off those tough times in our lives. Because of the harmful results, it's important to learn other ways to reduce stress so that fat is not used in this way. Much of our difficulty with fat is due to the way society sees it. We have to combat those commercials depicting the ecstasy of eating a chocolate bar. Having a chocolate bar is not really bad, but it's the images we associate in our minds that make it damaging to our way of life. Have you ever said, "I've had such a tough day that 'I DESERVE' that candy bar, piece of cake, or glass of beer?" Emphatically—it **is** important to find substitutes that can be used as a reward for the tough days we all have to deal with.

It would be nice if we borrowed some of the European eating philosophy of seeing dinner as an established ritual—a time to enjoy, with good food and good company. To their benefit, the Europeans aren't in such a rush and don't consume mass quantities of convenience, processed foods.

Food Cravings

Many people blame themselves for not being able to stay on a food program. The problem is not so much a matter of *will power* as it is conditioning for foods that create a system whereby the more they eat, the more they crave. For instance if you start off your morning with nothing or a doughnut and a cup of coffee with sugar, you probably have set yourself up for wanting more refined foods throughout the day. Refined foods taken into your system cause an impaired insulin response. That is to say, the pancreas secretes insulin to bring down the blood sugar level while the sugar is absorbed quickly, causing that spike of energy we all know and love. Unfortunately most of us can't maintain the sugar high. Due to the insulin, the blood sugar will drop way below its normal level so the brain is deprived of its sugar. You know you shouldn't eat those potato chips or candy bar, but your brain says *I want these things, because if I don't get some sugar soon, I'm going to pass out right here on the floor.* So your blood sugar rises again, you feel terrific, and the process is repeated many times throughout the day. Eating foods that are lower in fat and sugar and not so refined—fruits, vegetables, and fiber—will enable the food you eat to get into your system slowly to give you a good, solid, lasting level of energy. When the cravings are under control, it is the best feeling in the world because you are making your own choices, your body isn't making them for you. Your mind clears and makes good, solid, and wise decisions about what should fuel your body. You probably won't lose the craving for sugar altogether, but you will have it under control. Whoa, there's a piece of cake or an apple for me to eat, which will I chose? If you are in low blood sugar, the apple will be invisible, and you will take the cake because you need it. Learn to reevaluate that apple! Once those cravings are understood and under control, the rest of the nutritional elements can be implemented with relative ease!

Sugar & Kids

Our craving for sugar is not only learned as we are growing up, but it is inherent to our physical makeup. It's important, when raising children, to begin early to teach them that sweets are not the ultimate! They need to understand when they can have sweets. I'm not saying to deny kids cookies, but when you bring them into the house, don't stock up on five different types. Introduce small amounts of good quality cookies and cakes. Baking with the kids is an excellent way to get them started cooking (as early as three years old) and gives them a chance to eat their own creations. I recommend close supervision. Don't let young children too near the stove, but they can dig a little cup in a flour bag! They need to be exposed to cooking early so they can foster a healthy attitude about eating right. They need to understand what sugar does, and that it's not something for every day. If you bake yourself, you have more control over the ingredients you use, and you can pick the healthiest available.

Never use food or sweets as a reward or a punishment. Don't worry too much about what they like and don't like. If you introduce kids to carrots or other vegetables and they hate them, so what? They hate them. Introduce them again several months down the road. If they still hate them, wait another three months, they will probably learn to like them eventually. When I was a kid, and my mother will vouch for this, the only vegetable I would eat was canned cream style corn—no broccoli, no squash, nothing else. I'm living proof that food tastes can change as children become more sophisticated and understand why a balanced diet is so important.

Something to remember about sugar is that if you take in large amounts, the secreted insulin actually increases the fat in your body, so you gain weight. Though sugar and fat are different substances, they are usually related through their proximity in the sweets we love so much. Most people don't sit around and say, "I can't wait to have hard mints," they go for the fat in the brownies. I tell many of my clients that they don't have a *sweet tooth*, but what they really have is a *fat tooth*. The creamy-mouth feeling of fat greatly enhances our desire for sweet things. I've had many clients who have come in and shown me that they have been watching their fat intake, but they are still not losing weight. I usually find out that although the fat intake has indeed been reduced, they are still consuming a great deal of sugar. They don't realize that many of the fat-free, man-made products contain mass quantities of sugar. I recommend they cut the sugar out and guess what? They lose weight!

Goal Setting

Lifestyles of the fit and happy require a life plan. The list of written, definable, obtainable goals is a must. No one would set off to drive across the country without a road map, and that's what our lives need, a map of where we are and where we want to go. True lifestyle changes can be implemented gradually and piecemeal. Most people just don't think when it comes to their health. They only express a shallow desire to be better. Ask yourself—what do I want to accomplish five years out? Now, what part of that will I manage this year, the next, and the next? Not very many people can make all the changes they want all at once. It's much better to eat an elephant one bite at a time. For example, this year, "I will join a health club for exercise, lose X-amount of pounds, bring my cholesterol down, stop smoking, and have more fun in my life." OK, those are rather general goals. Now, break them down into goals for the next three months so you can be very specific about what you will do every day, week, and month. I make daily appointments with myself to exercise, because exercise is part of my plan. Left to my own devices, I know that, as important as exercise is to me, if I didn't write it down it wouldn't happen. When an idea is in some form of visual display, it is far more likely to be acted upon. I strongly suggest that people sit down with a piece of paper and a pen, or sit at the computer, and write down what they want to accomplish and by when. Be specific and make sure it's something that's challenging, yet can be accomplished. It shouldn't be so unrealistic that you can't get there.

For an example, I would like to tell a story about Beth, a very beautiful woman and a bit overweight. She had been working hard at eating all the diet products and watching her fat intake very carefully, but she wasn't exercising. She couldn't understand why she couldn't lose those extra pounds. I explained the relationship of exercise to diet and set up an exercise schedule for her. She now exercises every day and has lost 22 pounds. Her self esteem has soared! Her priorities were for everything and everybody else in her life. Now, her first priority is herself, and she is able to contribute much more to her company and her friends. She knows now that if she doesn't take care of her own personal needs, nobody else will.

Don't we ALL deserve to become the best that we can be?

The Right Atmosphere

Healthy dining and eating doesn't have to be green, brown, and bland. In fact, I believe that dining well, with exciting colors and shapes, together with fresh and interesting herbs and spices, is very important. Many diet programs de-emphasize flavor and texture, and I think that is a big mistake. I believe any program should offer an enjoyable experience in an atmosphere conducive to romantic or positive feelings.

My husband has painted our dining room so that the color is more exciting and produces a sense of wonderment. I think colorful place mats and real china and crystal heighten the experience of making dinner an event to look forward to and share with good company, whether it be family or that special someone. Low-fat food can be made to be very tasty and attractive without the feeling of deprivation. People can take time to eat and digest their food.

With this book, I challenge you to revive the art of dining and to have fun in the grocery store! I try to emphasize in every recipe that food should look interesting, appetizing, and flavorful. Today in our society most of our flavor comes from white foods—sugar, flour, and salt. When we take those away and substitute herbs, spices, and vinegars, we don't just throw flavor on top of the food and hide its true taste! If the food tastes good and clean, we will feel healthier just eating it. Once you get away from the sugar-laden processed foods, the apple will become a succulent, sweet, delicacy worthy of your palate. Train your sense of taste to appreciate the subtle nuances of food and enjoy the food itself. Seek quality, go to the bakery for breads, the butcher for meat, the farmers market for vegetables, and fish market for fish. Although food doesn't have to be expensive, this is not an area to scrimp and save, if you don't have to. Spend a little more time, money, and effort. It's worth it for a healthy and happy life.

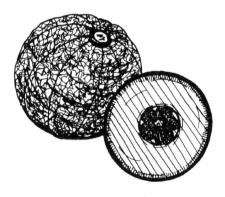

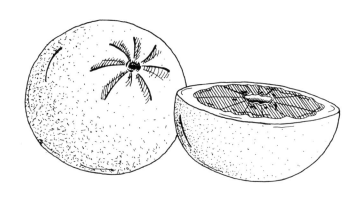

CHAPTER 2

The Importance of Water

Water is a forgotten nutrient and it's crucial to every function in the body. For example, it regulates temperature, conducts nerve impulses, and aids in circulation, metabolism, and eliminative processes. Water also boosts the immune system and other necessary body functions.

Dehydration occurs when you don't take in enough water to replace all that is lost through perspiration, respiration, urination, and other body processes. Dehydration reduces blood volume, which creates thicker, more concentrated blood. This may stress the heart and render it less capable of providing muscles with oxygen and nutrients and eliminating accumulated wastes.

You do not have to be perspiring profusely to lose water. You are losing it all the time. For instance if you are a frequent business traveler: your body could lose as much as two pounds of water in a three-to four-hour flight. Alcohol and caffeine, both diuretics, also increase the body's fluid loss. So does stress.

Drinking plenty of water prevents dehydration. Water helps regulate body temperature; promote smoother skin; keep bowel movements more regular and soft; increase resistance to infections by hydrating the mucous lining of the respiratory tract; and help prevent kidney stones, urinary infections, edema, and elevated blood pressure.

How much water do you need to drink? It depends on many variables including the foods in your diet, metabolic rate, weather, temperature, climate, physical activity level, and stress level. Here are some basic recommendations:

1. In general, drink between 6 and 8 cups of pure water every day, preferably between meals rather than with food.
2. Develop new water-drinking habits. Keep water accessible during the day and track your consumption. Put a glass of water next to you at work.
3. Sip beverages slowly.
4. Precede exercise sessions with extra water, generally 1 to 2 cups taken in the hour or so before training.

5. Consume more water immediately following exercise sessions and sports activities.

Getting used to drinking water is a habit you want to develop and integrate completely as an essential part of your life. Like any new health habit, it will take some time to readjust, but the results will be worth it.

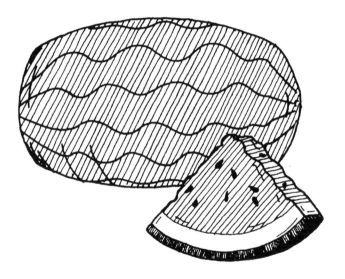

CHAPTER 3

How To "Just Do It"!

So, you *know* it's a good idea to work on your physical well being. Maybe it's the few extra pounds since high school, or a tired feeling as you mount the stairs, or for want of a few more reasons, you just can't ever seem to get started on a program and stick to it! If this isn't you, stay tuned anyway because whatever you want to start or stop doing, this is the way to *just do it.*

The first, and most important, in a series of questions that you must ask yourself is, *"What do I really want?"* Most people aren't sure of what they really want, but they are pretty sure they don't have it. So, how do you go about figuring out what it is that you really want?

Now, this is the hard part, take out a sheet of paper and a pen or pencil. Did you get that? Nothing—nothing—is going to happen for us until we take out that piece of paper and spell out for the mind what it is that we really want. When you write something on paper, it's nailed down and brings the mind into focus. This is the real **key**—the brain can define what it is that you want, so that the mind can focus on it and figure out how to get it. You don't have to figure out **how**, you just have to focus your mind on it. Let me re-emphasize, I'm trying to insist on the principal of "write it down." I know most people will never get past this first step, because it's just too easy!

Since most of us want more than one thing, write down several things on the "want" list. That's the way to set up some goals for yourself. Once you prioritize these things that you really want, single out the number one on your list. This is where we'll begin working.

Now for the purpose of this exercise, I am going to assume that the number-one goal is to improve your health by eating right and exercising. Remember, the process we are going to discuss can be used for anything you wish to achieve—whether it's to stop or start anything. To start loving, living, learning, etc., or stop smoking, worrying, fighting, etc. So, now you've written it down on a full size piece of paper—in big bold letters—as a symbol of what it is that you want enough to make a commitment to it. Take that master goal, break it down into doable chunks, and set time frames accordingly. The next step is to associate the pain/pleasure principle with the achieving of each aspect of the goal.

The only true motivators of the human will are pain and pleasure. Most of us spend all our lives moving away from pain and toward pleasure, never realizing that the real pain and pleasure connected with an act are seldom the same as those perceived. The actions we undertake to achieve what we really want will cause us pain and pleasure, but it's important to put into perspective the intensity and the value of each. So let's make a pain and pleasure chart for: **I want to improve my health by eating right and exercising.**

PAIN:

1. If I lose the extra pounds, nobody will notice or find me more attractive anyway.
2. I will have to fit exercise time into my busy schedule. My muscles will hurt and I will be stiff and sore.
3. Food won't taste good if it's healthy.
4. I won't have time to prepare healthy food.
5. If I start something, I don't know if I can finish it.

PLEASURE:

1. I will lose those pesky pounds and look more attractive.
2. When fit, I will feel better about myself and I will be more efficient.
3. My muscles will look toned and I will be a stronger person.

4. Healthy food will nourish my body properly.

5. Preparing healthy food will be fun and worthwhile.

6. If I start something and finish it, I will attain real self satisfaction.

You will have your own list. It's important to determine **all** the major forces of pain and pleasure associated with achieving goals.

Now we need to **question** the pain statements severely.

1. Do I really think no one will find me attractive?

2. How about me, myself?

3. Is it enough to look good in my own eyes?

4. I'll bet a special person will find me attractive.

5. Sure, my schedule is a busy one, but I'll bet I could make time in the morning by getting up a little earlier.

6. I'll bet when I feel better, I will be able to get more done in less time.

   No pain no gain, I'll bet with a little help from a personal trainer, I could learn a workout that would maximize gain and minimize pain. Well, I'm sure I will miss the fat and sugar in my diet, but what if I learn more about food and how to prepare it? I'll bet I would find food interesting and tasty. The same goes with time, I'll bet I can learn ways to prepare food that won't take so long. Get the picture?

Following the questioning of pain, we need to **intensify** pleasure.

1. How attractive will I look at my ideal weight?
2. I can see it in my mind's eye and I look marvelous.
3. I look fit; I feel good; how wonderful it will be!
4. My body will be toned all over and I will feel stronger and better about myself.
5. My body will function more efficiently when fueled correctly.
6. I will be able to get more done in less time than I ever did before.
7. I can see myself having fun in the kitchen preparing tasty, appetizing dishes in minimal amounts of time.

The gain is worth the pain specially when the pain won't be so bad anyway!

The third step is to REINFORCE THE COMMITMENT. What can we possibly do to make it difficult to fail? Can we tell someone close to us about what we have decided, so that they can gently chide us if we begin to stray from our path toward success? Maybe we can promise ourselves an irresistible reward for success or a despicable punishment for failure. I personally prefer the reward.

The fourth thing to do is CONFUSE the old pattern of behavior. If I'm in a hurry and am thinking about getting a fast burger, maybe I can begin to sing or hop on one foot. I need to do something, anything, that will take the focus away from the old way of doing things. This step is very important, because a body in motion tends to remain in motion and a body at rest tends to remain at rest! Without something to facilitate a change in our old behaviors, we will tend to continue doing the same old things.

The fifth step is to SUBSTITUTE a new, good behavior for an old, bad habit. Say you just love to have a candy bar whenever you are feeling stressed. You could substitute the desire for a candy bar with the desire for an apple. You could substitute going for a bicycle ride for watching TV in the early evening. With focus and determination you will be able to substitute positive activity for bad habits.

The sixth and final step is to ANALYZE your process. Is it working? Are you getting what you really want and achieving milestones toward your final goal? If not, it's probably because either your goal is not broken down into small enough increments or your process is flawed. If it is not working for you, go through the process again. Stress your reinforcement and renew your commitment, because if you are quite determined, you <u>can</u> "Just DO it!"

I WANT TO IMPROVE MY HEALTH BY EATING RIGHT AND EXERCISING!

Make a list of pain and one of pleasure.

Question pain.

Intensify pleasure.

Confuse old patterns of behavior.

Substitute new, good behaviors for old, bad habits.

Analyze the process.

Adapt, if necessary.

Just do it!

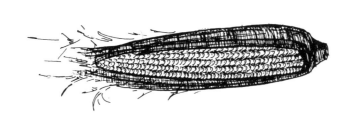

CHAPTER 4

Holiday Advice

Let's talk Turkey!

Yes, it seems that every time we turn around, it's holiday time again! For many that conjures up fears of how to handle the abundant array of tempting holiday foods that can easily deter the most vigilant dieter. During every holiday, it is my personal philosophy that one should enjoy oneself at the dinner table without doing too much damage to an eating program. Let's face it, the holidays are a hard time to stick closely to a weight-reduction program. The goal should be to get through this time without completely blowing the diet. Here are some hints to help you remain in control and make the holidays more enjoyable.

1. Establish a specific plan for what you will eat and what you won't. You will find yourself feeling less guilty if you planned for that piece of pie rather than denying yourself initially and then sneaking a piece or two later.
2. Get regular exercise. Don't let the holidays overwhelm you and disrupt your activity schedule. Also, make a plan to burn those extra calories you are bound to consume.
3. Don't starve yourself all day long in anticipation of the big meal. You will definitely overeat this way. Have a few light snacks throughout the day.
4. Try everything you want, just take smaller portions. It is sometimes easier to accept Aunt Minnie's stuffing with a smile, rather than go into a long rendition of why you shouldn't eat it.
5. Have a specific plan in mind to handle, IMMEDIATELY after the holidays, any excess weight gained or negative habits incurred.
6. Concentrate on enjoying family and friends and try to paticipate in non-food activities.
7. Go buy that smashing new outfit and remember to pamper yourself.

CHAPTER 5

TOP 10 Nutritional No-Nos

So many nutritional factors are said to be bad for us that we tend to think it is a good excuse to do nothing at all. The factors of sugar, fat, additives, cholesterol, and fast foods may seem overwhelming to manage. I've tried to simplify matters by listing my top No-Nos that deserve attention.

1. Eating without a plan or a goal: When you get in your car to drive somewhere, you have a destination or a goal in mind. But how many of us have a plan, a *road map*, for eating a healthy diet that will help us perform in the direction of our top potential? No matter how hard we try to navigate through the individual meals, our chances of following the right course day after day are poor. **Strategy for today**: Develop a healthy nutrition plan. Put some clear principles down in writing and post them in a highly visible spot, so you can follow your map.

2. Changing your habit too quickly: Change your diet slowly. Trying to make changes at 90 miles per hour will only cause you to crash. When you combine a gradual change with a sensible plan, you are bound to have a higher chance of success. **Action for today**: Write down a time frame for accomplishing specific parts of your diet plan. Be realistic.

3. Going longer than five hours without eating: After five hours without eating, you are subject to ravenous hunger and you do not care about health goals or good intentions. Biological rhythms and hunger stages are determined by our eating patterns. If people eat breakfast, lunch, and dinner in adequate amounts, appetite patterns will be established, and we will eat more regular meals. **Action for today**: Keep a food diary and identify your eating patterns.

4. Being in a *fat fog*: Excess fats are known to cause health problems. The adult diet should include an absolute maximum of 30 percent of calories from fat. Of the total fat grams only one third should be saturated. It is saturated fat in our diet that plays the most havoc with our health. **Action for today**: Begin to look at the fat content of all the foods you eat and actually visualize the amount of fat in one gram. One gram equals the weight of a standard paper clip! There are 9 calories per gram of fat. It's calories!

5. Skimping on produce and grains: Statistics from the United States Department of Agriculture (USDA) on food consumption show the average woman, age 19 to 50,

consumes only one cup of cooked vegetables and one medium fruit per day. We are eating too much fat and not enough complex carbohydrates. **Action for today**: Eat more vegetables, including dry beans and peas, more fruits and breads, cereals, pasta, and rice.

6. Being a member of the clean plate club: So many people clean their plates today because of the old messages they received as children. Today we need to eat based on our present needs, not on old tape recordings in our minds. **Action for today**: Examine your need to clean the plate. Instead eat based on your goals.

7. Trying to be too thin: Thin to look good and be reasonably trim is a sensible goal, trying to look like a fashion model isn't. **Action for today**: Recognize the body shape you inherited. Accept this shape and feed it a healthy diet.

8. Trying to lose weight without an exercise program: A low-fat diet that is combined with exercise protects lean body mass—metabolically active tissue—and promotes fat loss. Losing weight and keeping it off is tricky. Research continues to tell us that exercise is an important key to long-term success, but many people find it difficult to fit exercise into their schedules. If you are serious about losing weight and keeping it off, then you will have to reorganize your priorities and treat yourself to increased physical activity. **Action for Today**: Begin an exercise program you enjoy. Start slowly. Do just enough today, so you look forward to tomorrow.

9. Skimping on water: Because it is essential to so many body processes, adequate water must be available in the body at all times. On average, a total of two to three quarts of water are lost every day. Based on these losses, a minimum of two quarts of fluid should be consumed each day. **Action for today**: Make a conscious effort, each day, to drink one quart of water, one quart of other beverages, as well as high-water-content foods.

10. Giving food magical powers of bad and good: There is no doubt about it; a carrot is a healthier snack than a piece of candy! But snacks are only small components of your overall diet. The problem with categorizing all foods as good or bad is that it gives them a kind of power they really don't deserve. If you should eat a bit of food on your bad list, you may think of yourself as a bad person. Don't give food that much power to have control over your mind. **Action for today**: Recognize that you *can* eat most foods, but some are healthier than others.

CHAPTER 6

Thirty One Insights—One for Every Day of the Month

Thanks to Dr. David Kessler at the Food and Drug Administration (FDA), food manufacturers will have to follow more stringent requirements when it comes to the labeling of our food. We should expect to see some major changes in the upcoming year. People are becoming smarter as it relates to their own personal nutrition. The emphasis on overall fitness and health has replaced the emphasis on just losing weight quickly. Congress continues to investigate weight-loss scams and major weight-loss centers for their claims and credibility. And I think in the years to come these and other turn-arounds in the nutrition industry will continue to grow. In the mean time, here are 31 insights, one for every day of the month, to keep healthy, happy, and fit.

Day 1   The largest source of iron in the American diet is grain—notably, breads, pastas, and baked goods made with grain flour.

Day 2   One cup of cauliflower or broccoli contains more vitamin C than an orange and more than enough to meet the daily Recommended Dietary Allowance.

Day 3   Cooking in cast iron pots is a good way to increase the iron in your diet.

Day 4   Fig bars contain less than half of the calories and fat of most cookies, but twice as much fiber.

Day 5   Frozen yogurt made from whole milk can contain as much fat and sugar as ice cream. Make sure the yogurt is made from low fat milk and no fat is added.

Day 6   Singles tennis provides twice as strenuous a workout as doubles tennis.

Day 7   Children whose mothers smoke more than half a pack of cigarettes a day are twice as likely to have asthma.

Day 8   Since 1900 the percentage of Americans over 65 has more than tripled.

Day 9   Ground beef labeled *lean or extra lean* may actually contain up to 22% fat by weight, nearly as much fat as its regular counterpart.

Day 10   You would have to eat 32 cups of air-popped popcorn to get the 840 calories in a cup of oil-roasted peanuts. And to get as much fat in a cup of peanuts you would have to eat about 280 cups of popcorn.

Day 11   *Flavored seltzers* are usually calorie free, but a few now on the market contain sweeteners and thus have nearly as many calories as regular soft drinks.

Day 12   Cheap foods, costing less than 39 cents a pound, are generally healthy foods. That includes potatoes, bananas, carrots, rice, whole-wheat flour, and dried beans.

Day 13   More than 1,500 members of the U.S. Tennis Association are over 75 years old.

Day 14   A 200-pound person who starts walking a mile and a half a day and keeps on eating the same number of daily calories will lose on the average 14 pounds in a year.

Day 15   Minnesota, New Hampshire, and Utah have the healthiest populations, while Alaska, Mississippi, and West Virginia have the least healthy, according to a survey by Northwestern National Life insurance company.

Day 16   Eggs should not be stored in the egg section of the refrigerator door, since the temperature there is warmer than in the main compartment. Eggs should be stored in their carton in the coldest part of the refrigerator.

Day 17   Only 15% of the sodium in the American diet is added while preparing and eating at home. About 75% of the sodium comes from processed food. The remaining 10% is found naturally in food.

Day 18   A typical, plain 3.5 ounce doughnut has as many calories as four slices of bread with jam. Half the calories in a doughnut come from fat, but only 10% in bread and jam.

Day 19   The average Chinese blood cholesterol level is 127 milligrams per deciliter. The average American has a blood cholesterol level of 212 milligrams per deciliter.

Day 20   Vegetables generally lose 50% less minerals during steaming than boiling.

Day 21 The preference for sweet flavors appears to be inborn, but salt is an acquired taste. Many people placed on low-sodium diets change the threshold at which they can detect salt in their food after 6 to 8 weeks, even after eating salty foods from a young age.

Day 22 Ounce for ounce, raw green peppers have two and a half times as much Vitamin C as oranges, and red peppers have nearly four times as much.

Day 23 Japanese ramen noodles, packaged as the instant soup lunch in a mug, are very high in fat because they are usually dried by deep frying in lard or palm oil. Another drawback is the high sodium content of the seasoning packet.

Day 24 If you ever have a question about food safety, call the USDA's toll free Meat and Poultry Hotline at (800) 535-4555, weekdays, 10 a.m. to 4 p.m. Eastern time.

Day 25 Many flavored yogurts contain fruit jam, which adds the equivalent of eight or nine teaspoons of sugar per cup. The jam also takes up room otherwise filled by yogurt and its nutrients.

Day 26 Over time, smokers lose 20% to 30% more bone mass than nonsmokers. This results in a greater risk of fractures.

Day 27   Sweetened soft drinks usually contain 8 to 12 teaspoons of sugar in a 12-ounce can.

Day 28   A bacon cheeseburger has, on average, 250 more calories than a plain burger and plus a good deal more saturated fat and cholesterol.

Day 29   Don't store medication in the glove compartment of your car. The temperature there can be 50 degrees higher than outdoors, quickening the deterioration of the drugs.

Day 30   About 85% of food-borne illnesses could be avoided if consumers properly handled food.

31. Begin cooking for a lean life!

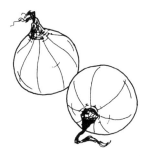

PART II

RECIPES

The Light Larder

There are a few things that I'd like to recommend that you keep on hand. If you are using some items that are not listed here, and they are low in fat, keep working with them. I'm sure they're fine.

For ease of categorization and discussion I've combined everything into three groups: *Seasonings*, *For the Refrigerator*, and *For the Pantry*.

The first area to deal with is seasonings—because it's crucial, crucial, crucial that low-fat cooking taste good! And we have to take out about everything that tastes terrific—like fat, which is a major source of flavor in our diet. The sweetness of sugar and savoriness of salt, also, are favorite staples of our diets. When you take out these three *whites*, something must be put back so that the belief that low-fat cooking has got to be boring, bland, brown, and green can be overcome. Seasonings will not only dispel that kind of thinking, but they will also add the color that is so important for eye appeal. To make foods taste good it's most important to use the most authentic spices available. There's no substitute for the real thing! Do not buy those *convenient*, packaged imitations of spices, juices, or garnishments. (Look in the appendix for all the brand names recomended.)

SEASONINGS

Fresh lemons and limes —Completely free of fat, citrus juices are a wonderful source of flavor! Using bottled lime or lemon juice just doesn't cut it. But you can have these juices readily available by extracting juice from fresh lemons and limes (any citrus fruit for that matter) using your microwave. Just throw them in a microwave-safe bowel, uncut, and cook about sixty seconds on the high setting. Let the fruit cool a bit (the skin will be hot), cut it in half and just hold it in your hand squeeze, and let the juice ooze out. Take that juice and freeze it in a freezer bag or plastic container. It will keep that way for several weeks.

Fresh herbs —Again, whenever possible, try to use fresh herbs and spices. The flavor is so much better, but if you just can't get them fresh, dried can suffice. You shouldn't be intimidated by the idea of trying to find them fresh; this can be extraordinarily easy.

For example, you can grow your own herbs and spices with just a box and some dirt! You can buy seed kits, some nurseries have them readily available. If you don't want to do that, it's OK, because most grocery stores now sell fresh, packaged herbs. If you do buy, don't just throw them, still in their little bag or box, in your refrigerator. I've seen them become completely dead after only a short time. Instead, take the herbs or spices and bundle them together with a string or rubber band. Put them in a glass of water and cover with a plastic bag. They will last about three days this way.

You also can freeze herbs in any sort of freezer bag or container. I recommend that you use these frozen herbs in something that you're going to cook. They do lose a little color and get a bit waterlogged. A stew or soup would be preferred instead of a fresh salad.

In a recipe that calls for dried herbs, always double the amount when using fresh. Cut them up, tear them, or use a food processor. You don't have to be fancy; you just need to get used to working with them because the resulting flavor is well worth the effort. The trouble with dried spices is that most people keep them in the cupboard for about ten years! I've been in some clients' cupboards and found boxes and bottles whose manufacturers have long since gone out of business. Shelf life on these things is about a year; so anything older than that, just toss it.

The most common herbs and spices that I suggest you have on hand are rosemary, basil, sage, chives, oregano, and dill.

Freshly ground black and white pepper —Rather than using pepper from the bottle, grind it! A plain old pepper mill is inexpensive; it doesn't have to be gold plated! Some of the clear plastic ones can be quite decorative when filled with multi-colored pepper corns.

Tamari soy sauce —This is a soy sauce with less sodium than the others and seems to have a more pleasingly, mild taste. It has salt—make no mistake about that, it's just less. For fancier dishes, try soy sauces in ginger, lemon, or garlic flavors.

Onions —For much more flavor and a little color, plain yellow onions can be replaced with shallots, scallions, purples, and Bermudas. Shallots are used extensively in Thai cooking, and you can usually find them in grocery stores. They are brown skinned and have a slight purple color with wonderful flavor.

Fresh ginger —The fresher the better! The skin should be tight against the flesh and it should almost shine. You don't have to buy a huge piece; you can break off just what you need. Never use powder, unless you are baking cookies or are desperate! It just doesn't provide the same kind of flavor. Fresh ginger will last about six months in the freezer and is actually easier to peel when it's frozen. Or you can keep it in the refrigerator for about two weeks. To use your ginger, peel the brown outer skin with a very good vegetable peeler and then chop or grate it. A ginger grater can be found in most oriental stores and will remove the little strings in the ginger as you grate.

Vinegars —More vinegars are available and are much more exciting than the widely used red wine or apple cider types. My favorites include balsamic, raspberry, and rice vinegar. The balsamic is very good with beans and salads. With its hearty taste and naturally brown color, it is used mostly in Italian cooking. The raspberry can be used with just about anything that calls for vinegar, and it is especially good with chicken. Sometimes when I'm lazy, I just throw chicken parts in the raspberry vinegar and let it marinate for about two days, then cook it on the grill. It's absolutely scrumptious that way! Vinegars can be kept at room temperature or in the refrigerator.

Mustards —Zero fat and good for low-fat diets any mustard is good.

FOR THE REFRIGERATOR

Low salt, low fat (1% milkfat) cottage cheese —If you like cottage cheese, be sure that it is 1% milkfat; 4% is a very high fat content. Be careful if you tend to load up on cottage cheese at the salad bar. It's probably the 4% variety, because that's much cheaper for restaurants to buy.

Part skim ricotta cheese —Use only 1 gram of fat or less per serving.

Whole grain breads —Here you really need dense, heavy, 100% whole grain breads, not wheat bread. It's nothing more than white bread with caramel coloring—light, spongy, and you can roll it up into a ball! I recommend that you go to a bakery or health food store to find your bread. (See the grocery list.) The difference is worth it.

Variety of vegetables and fruits —You may get real excited about cooking and want to stock up on everything you need to get started. Don't go overboard and buy too many fruits and vegetables at one time. Pick two or three vegetables for the week and use them during that week. Their nutritional value, vitamins and minerals, will simply be depleted while they sit in your refrigerator. It's a good idea to shop for your fruits and vegetables twice a week. For really fresh produce, try growing your own.

FOR THE PANTRY

Low sodium chicken broth or vegetable broth —Using a broth is a great way to cook when time is of the essence and taste is important. You can use it for marinating, sauteing, or just eating. If you don't make your own, I advocate finding a clear, low-sodium, low-fat broth, such as Health Valley. Most of the more popular brands, even though they say low sodium, are really high in sodium and fat. Bouillon cubes or granules are not recommended because of the high sodium content.

Low sodium canned tomatoes —During the winter when tomatoes aren't really their best, canned tomatoes such as Progresso can be very useful.

Salsa —Salsa, with its tomatoes and peppers, is high in Vitamin C and extremely low in fat. You also can make it yourself (recipe is in the book), if you'd like. If you'd rather buy it, I recommend Hot Cha Cha or Enricos.

Dry white wine —A basic Chablis or Chardonnay will suffice.

Dry sherry —Look for dry or very dry, but not sweet, after-dinner sherry. Many people seeing that a particular recipe calls for sherry, mistakenly buy what is referred to as cooking sherry. During prohibition it was loaded with sodium so no one would buy it to drink. Consequently, no one should buy it to cook with either! Buy the real thing.

Olive oil —Olive oil is the best oil to use for most of your cooking, because it's monounsaturated fat that can actually raise your HDL (good) cholesterol level. HDL is taken from the arterial walls for further reprocessing. LDL is the one that clogs the arteries. You know how you can remember which is which? LDL is lousy! Health aside, olive oil tastes the best, and you can use it for everything except baking. The greener the oil the more fruity and Italian. The yellower, the lighter it's going to be. If you don't use your oil a great deal, keep it in the refrigerator. It can become rancid in about six months if left out. Make sure you keep your olive oil in an opaque (can't see through) container, because it's very sensitive to air and light and the vitamins and minerals can be destroyed.

Sesame oil —Also monounsaturated, and a little bit goes a long way. The best way to use sesame oil is to add it after cooking. The flavor is so intense that when you cook or saute with it, your food will have that heavy taste. Dark sesame oil is more flavorful because the seeds are roasted a little longer, but most any kind is OK.

Vanilla extract —Important to have on hand if you bake. Get pure vanilla, not imitation.

No-sugar jams —I recommend Polaner All Fruit or Sorrell Ridge for those people who love sweets. Heated up, jam will make a delightful syrup for pancakes or ice cream.

Whole-wheat pastry flour —For those who feel that whole-wheat flour is just too heavy for their taste, whole-wheat pastry flour will improve the grain of your flour, while maintaining the lightness of white flour. You can use it in all your baking that calls for white or whole-wheat flour, except for yeast breads that will be too soft and will fall apart. Whole-grain flours will spoil, so its best to keep all whole-grain products in the refrigerator.

Oats —Oats are great for eating and baking.

Arrowroot —Used as a natural thickener, similar to corn starch. It's much better for making clear, clean looking sauces. Sometimes you will need a little more arrowroot than the corn starch called for in recipes. It is available in grocery stores, but I recommend that you buy it in bulk at a health-food store to save money.

→It does not need to Boil to thicken - Thickens at 180°*

Whole-wheat pasta —A good substitute for white pasta and a little heavier.

*graham kerr

Buckwheat noodles —Soba noodles, Japanese. Just take 5 minutes to prepare and toss with Tamari Soy Sauce and oriental style vegetables; it's delicious.

Brown and wild rice —I recommend short-grain rice because I think it tastes better and has a better texture. I do not recommend the quick cooking brown rices that are par-boiled so the vitamins and minerals have been destroyed. You are going to have to cook rice about fifty minutes, but I recommend you get a rice cooker that will do the job more easily and efficiently.

Bulgur wheat —A major ingredient in Tabouli salad, it is a Middle Eastern grain that cooks very quickly. It can replace rice and add variety to your cooking.

Lentils —Lentils are an alternative to rice and one of my favorite beans.

Herbal teas —Teas are wonderful hot or iced, depending on the season.

Sparkling waters —Be careful when buying water because some of the new sparkling/mineral waters, especially those with fancy names, have a great deal of sugar in the form of corn syrup. Don't buy those.

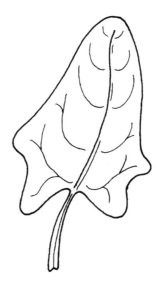

The Light Larder

(Tear out page and take it shopping!)

SEASONINGS

- Fresh lemons

- Fresh limes

- Fresh herbs (especially lemon grass, cilantro, basil, marjoram, chives, dill)

- Freshly ground black and white pepper

- Tamari soy sauce (low sodium variety)

- Onions (shallots, scallions, purple, bermuda)

- Fresh ginger

- Vinegars (balsamic, raspberry, bluberry, rice

- Mustards

FOR THE REFRIGERATOR

- Low salt, low fat (1% milkfat) cottage cheese

- Part skim ricotta cheese (look for 4 grams of fat or less) (Polly O Reduced Calorie)

- Whole grain breads

- Variety of vegetables and fruits

FOR THE PANTRY

- Low sodium chicken broth or vegetable broth (Health Valley is a good one)
- Low sodium canned tomatoes
- Salsa
- Dry white wine
- Dry sherry
- Olive oil
- Sesame oil
- Vanilla Extract
- No sugar, Jams
- Whole wheat pastry flour
- Oats
- Arrowroot
- Whole-wheat pasta
- Buckwheat noodles
- Brown and wild rice
- Bulgur Wheat
- Barley
- Lentils
- Herbal teas
- Sparkling waters

SPICY BEAN DIP
Ole! Ole!

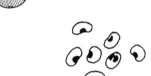

1 can pinto, kidney, or black beans, drained and rinsed
1 cup part-skim ricotta cheese or cottage cheese
1 Tbs cumin
1 Tbs chili powder
2 Tbs mild or hot salsa
1 jalapeno pepper, chopped
1 tsp fresh minced cilantro

Blend the beans with the rest of the ingredients and process until smooth.

This is a satisfying dip that can serve as a topping for a baked potato or even stuffed into pita bread. Serve with fat-free tortilla chips or pita bread wedges.

HUMMOUS
This recipe is practically fat-free!

1 15-oz can chickpeas, drain and reserve liquid or 1 cup chickpeas, cooked
3-6 garlic cloves
Juice of 1 lemon
Juice of 1 lime
1 tsp olive oil
Water

Place drained chickpeas in a blender. Add enough liquid to allow blender to mix the chickpeas. Add lemon and lime juice, oil, garlic, and rest of chickpea liquid to blend into a smooth consistency. Add up to 1/2 cup of water if consistency is still too thick. Hummous should be thick, but not sticky.

Commercial hummous recipes contain far more fat due to the addition of tahini (sesame paste, like peanut butter) and far more oil.

You can use hummous to top a baked potato or stuff into pita bread.

HERBED YOGURT DIP
Smooth and creamy for a baked potato or any vegetable!

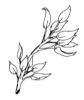

1 cup part skim ricotta cheese
1/2 cup yogurt, plain non-fat
2 Tbs low-fat mayonnaise
1 Tbs lime juice
1 tsp fresh chopped basil, dill or cilantro

Puree all ingredients in a blender until smooth.

Makes 1-1/2 cups.

HOT ARTICHOKE DIP

Traditional artichoke dip will blow your fat budget for weeks!
We cut out mayonnaise but left the flavor!

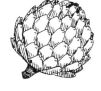

2 cans artichoke hearts packed in water (rinsed to reduce sodium)
2 cloves garlic
2 Tbs olive oil
1/3 cup lemon juice
1/4 tsp liquid hot pepper seasoning
1/4 cup grated fresh Parmesan cheese
2 cups finely ground whole-wheat bread crumbs (fresh bread, use about 1/2 of a loaf)
1/2 tsp minced oregano   1/4 tsp paprika
1/2 tsp minced basil   1/4 tsp minced thyme

In a blender or food processor, puree the first five ingredients for about 30 seconds. Pour the puree into a large bowl; stir in cheese, crumbs, and herbs. Transfer to an oiled 1-quart casserole.

Preheat oven to 350 degrees. Cover the dip and bake for 15 minutes or until slightly golden. Serve warm with whole-wheat crackers or breadsticks.

Makes 4 cups.

SHIITAKE MUSHROOM PATE
This recipe is great for party dips!

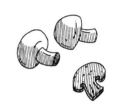

3 cups shiitake mushrooms, stemmed and sliced
2 Tbs broth (chicken or vegetable) or water
1-1/2 cups onion, chopped
1/2 cup fresh chopped green beans, cooked

Prepare mushrooms and set aside. Heat the broth in a skillet and saute onions until lightly browned. Add mushrooms; saute, stirring frequently, for 3-5 minutes, until just tender.

Transfer cooked mushroom mixture to a blender or processor and puree to a coarse grind. Add the green beans to the mushroom mixture and mix well. Chill before serving. Serve with crackers or spread on bread.

Tip: Do not wash your mushrooms! Mushrooms are a very porous vegetable. They will soak up the water you wash them with, then, while cooking, they will release their own moisture together with the excess water and you will have brown water on the bottom of your dish. Instead, take a paper towel or mushroom brush (looks like a nail brush) and gently dust off the dirt.

Makes 1-1/2 cups.

FIRST COURSE SHRIMP
Serve as a first course or as a main dish!

2 Tbs chicken broth
1 lb shrimp, peeled and deveined
1 tsp corn oil
2 scallions, minced
3 thin slices of ginger, peeled
2 garlic cloves, minced
3/4 cup chicken broth
3 Tbs tamari soy sauce

2 Tbs cider vinegar
1 tsp rice vinegar
1/4 tsp chili powder
4 tsp water
2 tsp arrowroot

Butter lettuce leaves
1/4 cup toasted sesame seeds

In a heavy skillet, heat the broth. Add the shrimp and saute for about 2 minutes. Remove shrimp and set aside. Add oil to the skillet. Add scallions, ginger, and garlic. Cook for one minute. Add broth, tamari, vinegar, rice vinegar, and chili powder. Mix the arrowroot with water and add mixture to the skillet. Stir for 2 minutes until sauce has thickened. Return the shrimp to the skillet and cook for 3 minutes. Pour mixture into a bowl, cover and refrigerate for at least 4 hours.

To serve: Arrange lettuce leaves on a platter and mound shrimp on top. Sprinkle with toasted sesame seeds.

Serve cold as in the recipe or hot. Substitute scallops, lobster, or crabs, if you like.

SESAME BASIL CHICKEN TIDBITS
This recipe is so nice for parties, but make a lot. You won't have leftovers!

4 chicken breasts, boned, skinned, and cut into cubes
1/3 cup tamari soy sauce
1 tsp olive oil
1 tsp sesame oil
4 dried red chilies or fresh chilies
1 Tbs sesame seeds
4 basil leaves, chopped

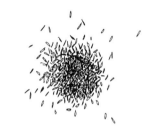

Combine all ingredients in a medium sized bowl. Let the chicken marinate for several hours (or even up to two days). Broil the chicken pieces for about 8-10 minutes, until cooked through. Serve with fancy toothpicks and additional tamari soy sauce on the side.

You may use the marinade for whole chicken breast filets, turkey fillets, thick pieces of fish—like salmon, tuna, swordfish, or shellfish.

Makes about 40 pieces.

RED PEPPER BRUSCHETTA
Pretty to look at, simple to make!

1 loaf Italian or French bread
3 garlic cloves, minced fine
1/4 cup olive oil

1/2 cup thinly sliced roasted red pepper
    (from the deli or make your own)
1/2 cup pitted black olives

Slice the bread into thin rounds. Combine the garlic and oil and spread over each piece of bread. Place the rounds on an ungreased cookie sheet in a preheated 375 degree oven. Toast until slightly brown. Top each round with a few pieces of red pepper and olives.

To prepare your own red peppers:
Place 3 or 4 peppers on your broiler pan and broil until they are completely black. Take them out of the oven and place in a resealable plastic bag. Let cool thoroughly. Rinse under cold running water to remove charred skin and seeds. You then have roasted peppers! Or you may spear one pepper at a time, hold over a gas flame and turn until blackened. Then proceed with above directions.

Rather than using slices you may puree the red peppers to make a paste. The amount of olives derived on each round is very little, so don't worry about your fat-intake!

Makes about 40-50 slices.

66 **SOUPS AND BREADS**—*Make a filling meal—simply!*

VEGETABLE STOCK

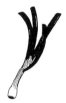

1 Tbs olive oil
2 carrots, coarsely chopped
2 celery ribs, coarsely chopped
1 large yellow onion, unpeeled, and coarsely chopped
1 leek, sliced (white part only)
1-1/2 quarts cold water
1 medium russet or white potato, peeled and chopped
3 fresh parsley sprigs
1 fresh thyme sprig
1 few black peppercorns

Heat the oil in a pan over medium heat. Add carrots, celery, onion, and leek. Cook, stirring, for 4 minutes. Reduce the heat to low, partially cover the pan, and cook the vegetables for 10 minutes until soft. Add all the remaining ingredients. Bring to a gentle boil. Reduce the heat to a simmer and cook, with the lid slightly ajar, for 2-3 hours. Strain the stock and pour into a quart sized container. Cook, cover, and refrigerate. It will keep for 3 days or for 3 months if frozen.

BASIC CHICKEN STOCK

4 lbs chicken backs and necks or a 4 lb chicken
4 quarts cold water
1 yellow onion, peeled and coarsely chopped
2 carrots, coarsely chopped
2 celery ribs, coarsely chopped
1 parsnip, cleaned and coarsely chopped

1 garlic clove, coarsely chopped
1 bay leaf
2 whole black peppercorns
1 fresh thyme sprig
4 fresh parsley sprigs

Wash chicken under cold, running water and place in a stockpot. Add cold water to cover. Slowly bring to a gentle boil. Skim the surface of the water as foam rises to the top. When the foam subsides, add all the remaining ingredients. Simmer, with the lid slightly ajar, for 2 hours.

Remove pot from the heat. Use tongs or a slotted spoon and remove the pieces of chicken. Strain the stock and pour into quart sized containers. Cool. Cover and refrigerate. The stock will keep in the refrigerator for 3 days. It may be frozen for later use.

Makes 3 quarts.

GAZPACHO
This is a chunky soup rather than the pureed version!

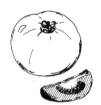

1 large cucumber
2 large tomatoes, seeded and finely chopped
1 large red or green bell pepper, seeded and finely chopped
1/4 cup fresh lime juice
3 cups chicken broth (defatted)
1 cup tomato juice
1 clove garlic, minced
1/2 cup sliced scallions
1 Tbs chopped fresh thyme leaves
1 tsp (or more!) liquid hot pepper seasoning

Peel cucumber and cut in half lengthwise; scrape out and discard the seeds. Finely chop the cucumbers. In a large bowl, combine the cucumber with the remaining ingredients. Season to taste with the liquid hot pepper seasoning. Cover and refrigerate for 4 hours or overnight.

If you wish, you may puree the vegetables, but do leave a few chunks—it gives the soup an interesting texture.

Makes 6-8 servings.

CHICKEN AND EXOTIC MUSHROOM SOUP
A warm, cozy soup for a cold, cold day!

1/2 lb chicken breasts, skinned and boned
1 Tbs tamari soy sauce
10 dried shiitake mushrooms
2 oz fresh porcini mushrooms, sliced
1 qt of chicken broth (low in fat and salt)

1 Tbs finely chopped scallions
1 Tbs soy sauce
1 Tbs sherry
Carrots, slices shaped with a vegetable
    cutter (optional)

Cut the chicken into 1/2 inch cubes. Soak the dried mushrooms in warm water for 20 minutes. Then drain and squeeze out excess liquid. Remove and discard the stems and finely slice the caps into thin strips.

Bring the broth to a simmer in a large pot. Add the dried mushrooms, fresh porcini mushrooms, scallions, soy sauce, and sherry. Continue to simmer the soup for 10 minutes. Add the chicken cubes and simmer together for 5-7 more minutes.

To each individual bowl, add 2-3 carrot slices that have been cut with a crinkle cutter. Pour soup over carrots.

You can substitute cooked shrimp, scallops, or shredded crab for the chicken.

Serves 4-6

SPANISH BLACK BEAN SOUP
Add additional spice, if you like!

2 tsp chicken broth
1 tsp olive oil
3 garlic cloves, minced
1 yellow onion, minced
1 tsp fresh minced oregano
1 tsp cumin
1 tsp chili powder or 1/2 tsp cayenne pepper
1 red pepper, chopped
1 carrot, coarsely chopped
3 cups cooked black beans (canned or from scratch)
1-1/2 cups chicken broth
1/2 cup dry red wine

In a large stockpot, heat 2 tsp chicken broth and 1 tsp oil. Add garlic and onions and saute for 3 minutes. Add oregano, cumin, and chili powder and stir for another minute. Add red pepper and the carrot. Puree 1-1/2 cups of the black beans in a blender or food processor. Add the pureed beans, remaining 1-1/2 cups of the whole beans, chicken broth, and red wine. Simmer for 1 hour. Taste before serving. Add additional spice, if you like.

Serves 6-8.

CREAM OF CARROT SOUP
So smooth and tasty!

2 Tbs chicken broth
3 Tbs finely chopped shallots or onions
2 Tbs unbleached flour
1 cup skim milk, scalded and hot
1 tsp cinnamon
1 cup cooked, pureed carrots or 2 cups pumpkin puree
1 cup chicken broth
Pepper to taste

Heat the broth in a stockpot over medium heat. Add shallots and cook until they are soft. Sprinkle with flour and cook for 2 to 3 minutes. Pour in hot milk and cook until mixture thickens. Add the remaining ingredients. Bring almost to a boil, stirring often. Add pepper to taste.

Makes 4 servings.

VEGETABLE SOUP WITH PASTA
Perfect for a cold winter's day!

1 Tbs olive oil
1 yellow onion, coarsely chopped
   or 2 shallots, minced
1 quart chicken broth
2 carrots, coarsely chopped
2 celery ribs, coarsely chopped
2 medium russet or white potatoes,
   peeled and cut into chunks

2 tomatoes, chopped
1 cup coarsely chopped escarole or spinach
1 tsp fresh chopped thyme
1 cup coarsely chopped yellow squash
1 bay leaf
2 tsp red wine vinegar
4 oz shaped pasta (corkscrews, shells, rigatoni)
Pepper to taste

Heat the oil in a saucepan over medium heat. Add the onion and cook, for about 7 minutes. Stir in the stock and the remaining ingredients. Simmer, covered, for 20 minutes, or until the vegetables are tender. Add the pasta and cook until pasta is done, about 9-10 minutes more. Remove the bay leaf. Add pepper to taste.

Makes 2 quarts.

JEANETTE'S CRANBERRY ORANGE SCONES

My assistant and right hand, Jeanette Van Winkle developed these wonderful scones that are great anytime. Typical scones have alot more fat than these.

1/2 cup dried cranberries	2 1/4 cups whole wheat pastry flour
2 Tbl honey	1 tsp baking soda
1/2 cup nonfat buttermilk, room temperature	1 tsp cream of tartar
3/4 cup orange juice	1/2 tsp. salt
Grated peel of one large orange	2 Tbs butter, cold

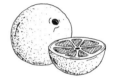

Preheat over to 375 degrees. Sprinkle a cookie sheet with flour.

Soak cranberries in boiling water for five minutes. Drain and set aside.

In a small bowl mix the honey and buttermilk, mixing well. Add orange juice and orange peel.

Sift flour, baking soda, cream of tartar and salt into a large bowl. Using a fork, or your fingers, cut in the two tablespoons of butter until well combined. Stir the buttermilk mixture and cranberries into flour mixture and mix gently by hand, until just combined.

Turn out the batter onto the floured cookie sheet and pat into a circle about 3/4 inch thick, 8 inches across. Using a sharp knife, cut the circle into eight wedges. Place pan into preheated oven and bake about 25 minutes.

Serve hot.

BANANA CARROT MUFFINS
A secret! Applesauce replaces the traditional fat!

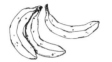

1-1/2 cups whole-wheat pastry flour
2 tsp baking powder
1 tsp baking soda
1/2 tsp nutmeg
Pinch of cloves
2 eggs or 1 egg and and an egg white

1/2 cup unsweetened applesauce
1/4 cup honey
1/2 cup buttermilk
1/2 cup mashed banana
1 cup grated carrot
1 tsp vanilla

Combine first five ingredients in a large bowl. Combine the remaining ingredients in a smaller bowl. Fold the two mixtures together. Spoon into non-stick muffin cups. Bake at 400 degrees for 20 minutes. Makes 2 dozen.

Variation: PUMPKIN MUFFINS - Omit the buttermilk. Substitute 1 cup of canned pumpkin and 1/2 cup chopped walnuts for the carrot and banana.

Applesauce may be substituted for oil, butter, margarine, or shortening—cup for cup—in ALL baked goods! However, with pie crusts, some fat is necessary and must be used to ensure a flaky crust.

SWEET POTATO AND ZUCCHINI BREAD

*A lovely way to combine sweet potatoes into a bread that is appropriate to serve at any meal.
Using applesauce instead of oil will considerably lower the fat content! And sweet potatoes are
an excellent source of vitamin A!*

2 cups whole-wheat pastry flour
1 tsp baking powder
1/2 tsp baking soda
2 tsp cinnamon
3 eggs (or 1 egg and 2 egg whites)
3/4 cup unsweetened applesauce

1/2 cup honey
1 tsp vanilla (or almond extract)
1-1/2 cups grated zucchini
1-1/2 cups grated sweet potatoes (or carrots)
1/2 cup chopped walnuts (optional)

Preheat the oven to 350 degrees. Lightly butter and flour a 9x5x3 inch loaf pan or bundt
pan. Combine the first four ingredients into a medium bowl. In a larger bowl, beat together
the honey, applesauce, eggs and vanilla. Mix in the zucchini and sweet potatoes. Add the
dry ingredients and walnuts and mix well. Transfer batter to the pan and bake in the oven
for 1 hour and 20 minutes. Cool bread in pan for about 15 minutes. Turn out onto a cake
rack and then let bread cool completely.

You can make muffins out of this recipe. Just raise the oven temperature to 425 degrees
and bake the muffins for 25 minutes.

Makes 2 dozen standard sized muffins.

HEALTHY COLESLAW
A much better version of the old standby!

1 cup yogurt, plain non-fat
1/2 cup wine or cider vinegar
2 Tbs honey
1-1/4 lbs cabbage, finely shredded (green and/or purple)
1/2 cup shredded carrot
1 Tbs caraway seeds or poppy seeds
1/2 cup raisins or currants

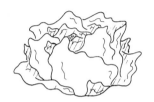

Combine yogurt, vinegar, and honey in a bowl. In a large bowl, add vegetables, caraway seeds and raisins. Toss with the dressing and serve.

Serves 6.

PENNE PASTA SALAD WITH BASIL VINAIGRETTE
Serve either warm or cold!

2 lbs plum tomatoes, cut into 1/2" cubes
1/4 cup olive oil
1/4 cup fresh chopped basil leaves
2 Tbs balsamic vinegar
Freshly ground pepper
1/2 cup chopped red onion
1/2 cup chopped roasted red bell peppers
1 lb penne pasta, cooked

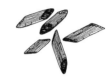

Combine tomatoes, oil, basil, vinegar, and pepper in a large bowl. Cook the penne pasta in boiling water until tender but firm, about 10 minutes. Drain. Combine the cooked pasta with the tomato basil mixture and add onions and peppers. Serve on a bed of lettuce.

Penne pasta is tube-like pasta that looks well with chunky sauces such as this one. Try to prepare this recipe when plum tomatoes are at their finest!

Serves 4

MIDDLE EASTERN TABOULI SALAD
My version has a lot less parsley!

1 cup bulgur wheat (raw)
2 cups boiling water
1 cup chopped parsley
3 medium tomatoes, chopped
1/2 cup chopped scallions or cucumbers
2 Tbs chopped mint
3 Tbs lemon juice
2 Tbs olive oil
1/2 tsp pepper
1 tsp cumin

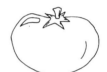

Place bulgur in a medium heat-proof bowl. Bring 2 cups water to a boil and pour over the wheat. Let stand for at least 1 hour to plump grains. In a large bowl, combine bulgur with parsley, tomatoes, scallions, mint, olive oil, and lemon juice. Toss to mix well. Season with pepper and cumin.

Although I like parsley, I think too much of it can give the salad a *grass*y taste. This salad is nice to have any time!

Serves 6-8

QUINOA SALAD

1 cup quinoa, cooked (or couscous)
1/4 cup finely chopped red or yellow pepper
1/4 cup finely chopped carrots
1/4 cup finely chopped celery
2 Tbs finely chopped Italian parsley

Lots of freshly ground pepper
1 Tbs olive oil
4 Tbs rice vinegar
2 garlic cloves, minced
3 Tbs finely chopped scallions

Combine the quinoa with all the vegetables. In blender combine oil, vinegar, garlic, scallion and pepper. Blend. Pour over the quinoa and serve.

Makes about 4 servings.

QUINOA (pronounced keen-wa) is a wonderful grain. It is very high in protein and is simple to prepare. All you do is rinse it well in a fine strainer (to remove the bitterness) and cook it in double the amount of water for 15 minutes. You can purchase quinoa in gourmet and health food stores.

COUSCOUS, also known as Moroccan pasta, is also very simple to prepare. Pour double the amount of water over dry couscous in a heatproof bowl. Let it sit 5 to 10 minutes, until all the water is absorbed. Finished! You can purchase couscous at gourmet and health food stores and some major supermarkets.

BLOOD ORANGE SALAD WITH ROMAINE AND KIWIS
A deep rose, picture-perfect salad, with full flavor!

1 head romaine lettuce torn into small pieces
3 kiwi fruits, peeled and sliced
2 blood oranges, peeled and sliced
3 Tbs apple cider vinegar
1 tsp fresh lemon juice
1/4 tsp freshly ground pepper
2 Tbs walnut oil
1 small red onion, sliced into rings

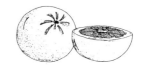

Wash the lettuce and gently tear into small pieces. Prepare the fruits. In a small bowl, combine vinegar, lemon juice, pepper, and oil. Arrange the fruits and kiwis over the lettuce on a serving platter and place the onion rings on top. Drizzle the dressing over all.

When you can get them, blood oranges are one of the most beautiful fruits to look at! They give this salad its unusual appeal.

Serves 4-6

BLACK BEAN JICAMA SALAD

Jicama, the Mexican potato, is one of my favorite vegetables. It is a brown skinned vegetable that ranges in size from small to large. To use, just peel the skin off and cut slices. It has a texture like a water chestnut, is slightly sweet, and is low in calories. It is my personal promise that this salad will disappear from everyone's plate fast, so make a lot!

3 cups cooked black beans (canned, rinsed, and drained, or from scratch)

2 tomatoes, chopped

2 red peppers, finely chopped

3 garlic cloves, minced

3 jalapeno peppers, chopped (remove the seeds if you want to)

1 Tbs cumin

1/4 cup fresh lime juice

1 Tbs red wine vinegar

1 Tbs olive oil

1 cup diced jicama

1 cup yellow corn (off the cobb or frozen)

2 Tbs fresh chopped cilantro

Combine all the ingredients and let them sit in the refrigerator several hours to blend the flavors.

Makes 8 servings.

COLORFUL LENTIL SALAD
Very filling and the flavor improves with time!

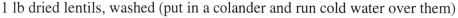

1 lb dried lentils, washed (put in a colander and run cold water over them)
3 cups water

2 large green peppers, cored, seeded, and diced   2 Tbs olive oil
2 large red peppers, cored, seeded, and diced   2 tsp cumin
2 large cucumbers, peeled, seeded,and diced   1/2 tsp dried oregano or 1 tsp fresh oregano
3 stalks of celery, diced   3 Tbs lemon juice
1 red onion, diced   1/2 tsp black pepper
2 cloves of garlic, minced

In a large saucepan, bring the lentils and water to boil over high heat. Reduce the heat to low, cover, simmer for 35-40 minutes. Drain and set aside.

In a large bowl, mix together the oil, lemon juice, cumin, oregano, and pepper until well blended. Add the lentils and vegetables. Cover and marinate in refrigerator. Will keep up to three days. You can use other beans, if you wish—kidney, pinto, white or black beans.

Serves 6-8.

WILD RICE SALAD
A nice hearty salad that has a slight sweet flavor

1 cup raw wild rice
4 cups cold water
1 cup mandarin oranges, packed in their own juice,
　　drained and reserve 2 Tbs juice
1/2 cup chopped celery
1/4 cup minced red pepper
1 shallot, minced
1 tsp mined thyme
2 Tbs raspberry vinegar
1 Tbs olive oil

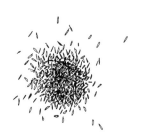

Prepare the rice. Rinse the raw wild rice with cool water in a sieve until the water is clear. Place the raw rice and the 4 cups of water in a saucepan. Bring to a boil, lower the heat, and cover the pan tightly and let it cook for 45-50 minutes until the rice has absorbed the water. Set the rice aside to cool.

In a large bowl combine the mandarin oranges (remember to reserve 2 Tbs of the canned juice), celery, red pepper, and shallot. In a small bowl, combine the reserved juice, thyme, vinegar and olive oil. Add the rice to the mandarin oranges and pour the dressing over the salad. Serve.

Makes 4-6 servings.

ORIENTAL TURKEY SALAD

Here's a recipe utilizing leftover turkey you could pull from the bird or buy turkey fillets, cook them, and slice into strips. The recipe is perfect for pieces of meat that have become dried out. The secret is in the dressing!!!

2 cups sliced leftover turkey or 1 lb turkey fillets, cooked and sliced into strips
2 cups sliced celery   1/2 cup minced scallions
1 cup fresh snow peas, stems removed   1 cup cooked soba noodles
1/2 cup red pepper, diced

Dressing:
6 Tbs plum vinegar (sold in gourmet, health, and Oriental grocery stores)
1 tsp sesame oil
1 tsp honey   1/4 tsp white or black pepper
2 tsp sherry (dry)   Romaine lettuce leaves
2 cloves garlic, minced   Sesame seeds

Toss in the turkey with the vegetables and soba noodles in a large serving bowl. Combine all dressing ingredients. Pour dressing over the turkey salad. To serve: line plates with lettuce leaves, top with some of the salad. Garnish with sesame seeds.

Makes 4 servings.

HOW TO PURCHASE CHICKEN

Some people think chicken is chicken is chicken! There are a few steps you should take to purchase and prepare chicken.

If you can, try to purchase organic chickens which were allowed to roam free rather than being penned up in a small cage. Their meat is more tender and less fatty. It is a real treat if it is available to you. Price-wise it really is not that much more than regular chicken and the taste is worth it.

I will give the directions for purchasing chicken breasts, since the breast meat is lower in fat than the dark meat. You should try to purchase chicken breast with the skin left on and bone removed. The skin will keep the chicken from drying out before you cook it and your final product will be much more moist. There is additional fat that is removed when the bone comes off, so try to get chicken boneless. Do not, however, eat the skin! It contains 40 grams of fat per 3-1/2 ounce serving! I leave the skin on up to when I am ready to cook.

Wash the chicken in cool water and pat dry. Chicken should be handled with clean knives and a clean cutting board. I keep a separate cutting board just for poultry. The jury is still out on whether a plastic or wooden board is better! I still use a heavy plastic board that cleans up beautifully in the dishwasher. Make sure you thoroughly clean knives, boards, and your hands after handling raw poultry.

Avoid defrosting and then refreezing chicken. The texture becomes very rubbery and distasteful. See the refrigerator and storage charts in this book for storage of chicken.

Use methods of cooking chicken that seal in the flavor. Avoid the practice of putting a chicken breast under direct heat. Please cook all chicken thoroughly. Chicken is done when no pink color remains. Remember, it is not vogue to eat pink chicken! The following recipes help to keep chicken delightfully moist. Enjoy!

HOW TO BUY FISH

Fresh Fish: When you buy whole fish, look for bright, clear eyes, red gills, and bright tight scales or shiny skin. Stale fish have cloudy, sunken eyes; with age, gill color fades to light pink. The flesh should be firm and springy. Fresh fillets or steaks should have flesh that appears to be freshly cut, without a dried or brown look, and should be firm in texture.

Frozen fillets: Wrapping should be of moisture-vapor proof material with little or no odor. Look for solidly frozen flesh with clear color, free of ice crystals. Discoloration, a brownish tinge, or a covering of ice crystals all indicate that the fish may have been thawed and refrozen.

HOW TO STORE FISH

Fresh: Keep fresh fish and shellfish loosely wrapped, in the refrigerator, and cook within one day.

Frozen: Keep in the original wrapper; use immediately after thawing. Never thaw and refreeze fish, since this will cause moisture loss and texture and flavor changes.

HOW TO THAW FISH

The best way to thaw frozen fish is to leave it in its wrappings and thaw it in the refrigerator or in cold water. Thawing at room temperature can cause sogginess. Drain well and blot dry with paper towels.

HERBED CHICKEN
The aroma—aah!

About 3 lbs chicken breasts, boned and skinned
Freshly ground pepper
2 Tbs parsley (Italian)
2 tsp fresh thyme
2 tsp fresh rosemary
4 sage leaves
1 tsp fresh tarragon
1/4 cup olive oil
2 Tbs sherry vinegar

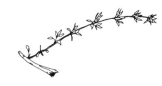

Place the chicken breasts in a baking dish. Sprinkle each one with fresh pepper. In a blender or food processor place remaining ingredients. Blend until smooth. Pour the herb mixture over each breast.

When ready to cook, preheat the oven to 350 degrees. Bake for 35 to 45 minutes until chicken is cooked throughout. Try not to dry chicken out, use a little white wine to baste if necessary.

Make sure the herbs are fresh. That makes all the difference!

Makes 4-6 servings.

CHICKEN SAUTE WITH VEGETABLES
Very tasty and healthy, too!

2 whole chicken breasts, halved,
  boned, and skinned
1 egg white
1 Tbs arrowroot
2 Tbs water or chicken broth

1/2 cup sliced Shiitake mushrooms (fresh or dried)
2 small zucchini, cut into strips
1 cup fresh snow peas, trimmed
1 Tbs tamari
1/4 cup sliced scallions

Flatten each piece of chicken: place between 2 sheets of waxed paper and pound it with a mallet until it is about 1/4 inch thick. Cut into bite-size pieces. Place chicken in a medium size mixing bowl. Add the egg white and stir until the chicken is coated. Stir in the arrowroot thoroughly. Let sit for about 10 minutes, then place in a large heated skillet with the water or broth. Saute, stirring occasionally, just until the chicken is opaque throughout.

Remove chicken from the skillet. Add mushrooms to the pan and stir over medium heat until they begin to release their liquid. Add zucchini, scallions, snow peas, and tamari. Cook over medium heat, stirring frequently, until vegetables are crisp and tender. Stir in the chicken and heat through.

Serves 6.

LEMON CHICKEN
A delicious alternative to the very sweet traditional lemon chicken!

1 lb chicken breasts, skinless and boneless
2 egg whites   1 Tbs corn oil
4 tsp arrowroot   1 Tbs chicken broth

Sauce:
2/3 cup chicken broth   4 Tbs fresh lemon juice
3 tsp honey   1 tsp tamari
2 tsp sherry
1/2 tsp finely chopped garlic   2 tsp arrowroot
1/2 tsp chili powder   2 tsp water

Cut chicken into strips 3 inches long. Combine with egg whites and arrowroot in a bowl. Chill chicken for about 20 minutes in the refrigerator. Heat the oil and broth in a wok until it is moderately hot. Add the chicken strips and stir quickly. Remove chicken and drain on paper towels. Wipe the wok clean and add all the sauce ingredients except the arrowroot and water. Bring to a boil. Combine arrowroot and water and add to sauce ingredients. Lower the heat and simmer for 1 minute. Return the chicken to the skillet and stir-fry 1 minute more.

Serves 4-6.

WILD RICE SUN DRIED CHERRY STUFFED CHICKEN

4 whole chicken breasts, halved, skinned and boned
Freshly ground pepper

Stuffing:
2 cups cooked wild rice (about 1 cup raw, follow package directions)
1/2 cup rehydrated sun dried cherries (available at gourmet stores) or cranberries
3 Tbs vegetable or chicken broth
1 shallot, minced
1/4 cup minced celery
2 tsp minced fresh rosemary
3/4 cup dry white wine
Paprika

Prepare chicken: with a meat mallet, pound the breasts to a 1/4 inch thickness or buy already pounded fillets. Sprinkle pepper over each half. Set aside.

Prepare stuffing: Cook rice according to package directions. If you make too much rice, never fear! Just double the stuffing recipe and serve as a vegetarian meal. The stuffing will keep fresh for 1 week. Rehydrate the cherries. In a skillet over medium heat, saute the shallot and celery in the broth. Add the rosemary. Add the vegetable mixture to the rice and toss in the cherries.

To assemble: Using a flat surface, spread the chicken breasts out for rolling. Use a few spoonsful on one end of the chicken breast and roll until the stuffing is completely encased with the ends tucked under. Secure with a toothpick. Repeat the procedure with each piece of chicken. Place the rolled breasts in a casserole and sprinkle liberally with paprika. Pour white wine around the breasts in the casserole.

Cover and bake at 350 degrees for 35-40 minutes. Remove the cover during the last 10 minutes of cooking time.

Makes 6-8 servings.

Any leftover stuffing? Place in a casserole and bake, covered, for 30 minutes. Good, as is, or use to fill acorn squash, peppers, eggplant, or zucchini!

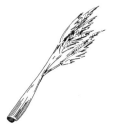

GRILLED CHICKEN BREASTS WITH SALSAS
Fabulous!

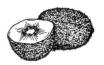

4 whole skinless, boneless, chicken breasts
Olive oil for brushing the chicken with tomato salsa
Sesame oil for brushing the chicken with fruit salsa
Salsas
Lime wedges for the tomato salsa
Kiwi slices for the fruit salsa

Preheat broiler or grill. Brush the chicken breasts with either olive or sesame oil and broil or grill about 5-6 minutes per side or until no pink remains.

To serve: Place salsa of choice on a plate using a few spoonsful per person, top with a chicken breast, and garnish with either a lime wedge or kiwi slice.

Makes 6-8 servings.

FRUIT SALSA

1 ripe pineapple, peeled, cored, and chopped into chunks or 2 cans water-packed
pineapple chunks   1 Tbs minced red pepper
1/4 cup white vinegar (only with fresh pineapple)   2 Tbs rice vinegar
1 mango, peeled and cubed   1 Tbs finely minced cilantro
1/2 papaya, peeled, cubed (use remaining half for papaya mousse recipe in this book)

If using fresh pineapple, cook the chunks in the white vinegar for 15 minutes until softened. Set
aside to cool. If using canned pineapple, combine the pineapple with the other ingredients and
let steep an hour or two. As soon as the fresh pineapple has cooled, follow the above directions.

SALSA
Wonderful with anything and everything!

6 medium tomatoes, seeded, and chopped   1/2 cup finely chopped onions
1/4 cup chopped fresh parsley   2 Tbs chopped fresh cilantro
2 long green, mild chili peppers, seeded (or 1 jalapeno, seeded and chopped)
1 Tbs red wine vinegar   1 garlic clove, minced
1/2 tsp fresh oregano

Combine all ingredients and chill for 1 to 2 hours.

Note: Leave the seeds in the jalapenos if you want a *hot* salsa.

HONEY-LIME-TEQUILA CHICKEN

A little bit of the islands brought to your kitchen! Great dish for parties, a luau perhaps?

4 chicken breasts, skinned and boned

Marinade:
2 Tbs honey
2/3 cup fresh lime juice
1/4 cup tequila
2 cloves garlic, minced
1 yellow onion, minced
1 red pepper, minced

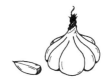

Combine marinade ingredients and pour over the chicken breasts. Marinate for at least 1 hour. Drain the marinade and grill on each side about 7-8 minutes per side or until no pink remains.

Makes 6-8 servings.

OVEN FRIED CHICKEN
Serve with your favorite tomato sauce!

4 large whole chicken breasts—skinned, trimmed of fat, and halved
1/2 cup whole grain cracker crumbs (place crackers in blender and crumb)
    (AK-MAK, Health Valley Herb, Ryvita are good.)
1/2 tsp black pepper
1 tsp onion powder
1 tsp garlic powder
1/2 tsp thyme, dried or 1 tsp fresh
1/2 paprika
1/2 tsp oregano, dried or 1 tsp fresh
Tomato sauce

Combine all ingredients except chicken. Shake or roll chicken in the crumb mixture. Place chicken in a large 9" x 13" baking pan. Bake uncovered for 35-45 minutes, until well browned.

Makes 4-8 servings.

ITALIAN TURKEY STIR FRY

Another use for leftovers! This time turkey is jazzed up Italian style with ingredients you probably keep on your cupboard shelf!

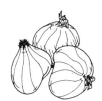

2 Tbs chicken broth
1 clove garlic, minced
1/4 cup dry white wine
1 tsp chopped fresh oregano
2 tsp chopped fresh basil
1 cup your favorite tomato sauce
1/2 cup fresh parsley leaves (Italian, if you can find it)
1 Tbs capers
1 Tbs minced black olives
2 cups leftover turkey, cut into strips or 1 pound of turkey fillets, cooked and cut into strips

Heat the broth in a wok or skillet over medium-high heat. Saute the garlic for a few minutes until lightly browned. Add wine, oregano, and basil. Cook for about 10 seconds. Add the tomato sauce and cook a few minutes more. Add the parsley, capers and minced black olives. Add the turkey to the skillet and heat thoroughly.

Makes 4 servings.

WHITE FISH PATE
What a wonderful way to use leftover fish!

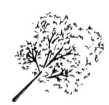

1/2 cup 1% cottage cheese or 1/2 cup part-skim ricotta cheese
1 Tbs Dijon mustard (grainy or smooth)
1 tsp fresh chives
1 tsp fresh dill
1 tsp fresh parsley
1/4 tsp white pepper or black pepper
Dash tamari soy sauce
1 cup leftover cooked flounder or any white fish

In a blender, combine all ingredients except the fish. Add the fish and mix in by hand. Chill covered for two hours before serving. Serve with crackers or breadsticks.

Sometimes we just don't know what to do with leftovers and this fits the bill! Put into a nice crock and serve on any buffet.

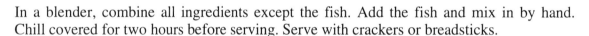

WHITE FISH IN FOIL
A simple, simple way to prepare fish!

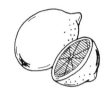

1 whole trout or bass
Freshly ground pepper
1 cup soft bread crumbs (make from whole wheat bread,
    place approximately 1/4 loaf into a food processor or
    blender and crumb)
2 tsp olive oil
2 tsp chopped dill
1 small onion, chopped

Prepare your outside grill or inside broiler by placing the rack six inches from the coals or the broiler rack six inches from the heat source. Rinse fish inside and out with cool water and pat dry. Combine the bread crumbs, oil, dill, and onion together. Stuff the cavity of the fish with the bread stuffing. Oil a sheet of heavy duty aluminum foil and wrap the fish tightly in the foil. Grill fish for about 30 minutes, turning once or twice. The fish will be mildly flavored and moist.

If you're pressed for time, your fish market can clean and trim the fish. Then there is no clean-up time for you!

Serves 4–6

SEAFOOD KEBABS HAWAIIAN
Fun to eat!

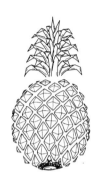

1/2 cup sherry
1 Tbs sesame oil
2 Tbs grated fresh ginger
1 Tbs tamari soy sauce
2 Tbs pineapple juice concentrate
1 lb fresh scallops or shrimp
1 lb fresh ripe pineapple, cut into 6 wedges
1 mango, cut into 6 large wedges
1/2 papaya, cut into 6 large wedges
1 large red pepper, seeded and cut into 1" squares

Combine the first five ingredients in a medium bowl. Add the scallops or shrimp. Marinate at room temperature for 30 minutes. Prepare a hot fire or oven broiler. Remove scallops or shrimp from the marinade and pat dry. Reserve the marinade. Thread the seafood onto 6 long metal skewers, alternating with pineapple, mango, papaya, and red pepper. Grill over hot coals, for about five minutes.

If you would like to use wooden skewers, be sure to soak them in warm water for 15 minutes before threading on the food. You can use any vegetables, such as whole cherry tomatoes, pieces of corn, zucchini chunks, or whatever!

Makes 6 kebabs.

RED SNAPPER VERACRUZ
Cinnamon with fish, you say? It's delicious!

3 tsp olive oil
1 small green pepper, chopped
1 medium onion, chopped
3 cloves garlic, minced
1/4 tsp ground white pepper
1 tsp cinnamon
Juice of 1 lime
1/4 cup canned green chilies
3 large tomatoes, seeded and coarsely chopped
4 red snapper or rockfish fillets

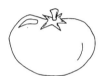

Heat the oil in a large skillet over medium-high heat. Add pepper, onion, and garlic; cook for about 7 minutes. Add the white pepper, cinnamon; cook for one more minute. Add the tomatoes and bring the mixture to a boil; cook until thickened (about 5 minutes).

Place the fillets in a lightly oiled baking dish. Pour sauce over the fish and bake at 350 degrees until fish is slightly translucent—about 10-15 minutes.
This authentic dish treats fish right!

Makes 4 servings.

ELEGANT COLD SALMON WITH DILLED CUCUMBER SAUCE
This method of cooking is what I term "oven poaching!"

3 salmon steaks or thick slices from salmon fillet (skin removed)
1 Tbs fresh lemon juice   Shredded blanched purple cabbage
6 cherry tomatoes   Romaine lettuce leaves
Dilled cucumber sauce (see recipe)

Cut each salmon steak vertically in half, removing the bone and skin. Rub each piece with a little lemon juice. Wrap a salmon slice around each cherry tomato. Wrap each piece in plastic wrap and arrange in a dish with 1" water. Bake at 325 degrees for 20 minutes.

Hold cooked salmon in refrigerator until cooled. To serve: place romaine lettuce leaves and shredded blanched purple cabbage on each plate. Unwrap salmon and add the cooked salmon on top of the cabbage. Pour a thin layer of the dilled cucumber sauce on top.

Use a very good quality of plastic wrap. When wrapping the salmon, fold the ends over to tightly seal the piece. Make sure you remove the wrap only after the fish has cooled. You can get burned handling hot plastic wrap!

Note: To blanch cabbage: boil 3 cups water in a medium saucepan. Add 1 cup cabbage, coarsely chopped. Turn off heat. Drain cabbage. Rinse cabbage with cool water and pat dry. This method helps the cabbage to retain its nice purple color.

Makes 6 servings

DILLED CUCUMBER SAUCE
Serve over salmon or any vegetables. Delightful!

1 cup non-fat plain yogurt
1/2 cup chopped, seeded cucumber
1 tsp cider vinegar
1 tsp fresh dill
1 tsp fresh chives

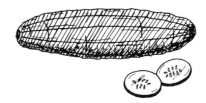

Combine all ingredients.

Makes 1-1/2 cups.

CALIFORNIA FISH SALAD
Quite a change from tuna salad!

1 lb fish steaks, cooked (Swordfish, Mahi-Mahi, Salmon, Halibut, cooked in any fashion)
1 large onion, chopped
Juice of 2 limes
1 red pepper, chopped
1 Tbs olive oil
1 Tbs chopped jalapeno peppers
1 Tbs chopped fresh cilantro
4 ripe tomatoes, cut into wedges
Hydroponic lettuce leaves or other dark lettuce
Lime wedges and fresh cilantro for garnish

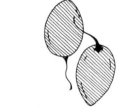

Break fish into bite-size pieces, removing any bones. In a medium bowl, combine all ingredients except the tomatoes and lettuce leaves. Chill until ready to serve. Arrange lettuce on salad plates. Spoon fish salad onto center of plate. Surround with tomato wedges and garnish with lime wedges and cilantro.

Use as a main meal or as an appetizer.

Makes 4 servings.

NEW ORLEANS SHRIMP CREOLE
Enough for a party AND the possibilities are endless!

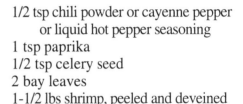

1/4 cup dry white wine
2 cups diced onions
1 cup diced celery
1-1/2 cups diced green and red peppers

2 tsp garlic powder
1/2 cup okra, sliced (try to get it fresh)
2-1/2 cups plum tomatoes, diced OR
    1-1/2 cups canned Italian plum tomatoes, crushed
1 Tbs low-sodium tomato paste
1/2 cup chicken broth

1/2 tsp chili powder or cayenne pepper
    or liquid hot pepper seasoning
1 tsp paprika
1/2 tsp celery seed
2 bay leaves
1-1/2 lbs shrimp, peeled and deveined

Place wine in a large pot; bring to a boil. Add peppers, onion, and celery. Saute for 10 minutes. Add remaining ingredients, except the shrimp. Lower the heat and simmer for 45 minutes. Add the shrimp and simmer 5-7 minutes longer.

This recipe has many uses. You may substitute shrimp, crab, scallops, lobster or pieces of fish, like haddock or halibut. Add at the end and let simmer 5-8 minutes longer. You can make the base and, before adding fish, freeze it for 6 months!

You can use the base over pasta, rice, or potatoes. You can add clams or mussels, cover and let steam until the shells open.

CHINESE ORANGE FISH
A quick and easy dinner!

5 Tbs vegetable or chicken broth
1 lb rockfish, orange roughy, OR
    bass, skin removed and cubed OR
        1 lb shelled and deveined shrimp
1 garlic clove, minced
1 shallot, minced
1/2 cup chopped red pepper
1/2 cup sliced celery

1 cup fresh snow peas, trimmed
1/2 cup sliced water chestnuts
1/2 cup fresh orange juice
1 Tbs arrowroot
1 tsp sesame oil
1 tsp rice vinegar

chopped scallions for garnish

Heat 3 Tbs of broth in a wok or heavy skillet. Add the fish and, over high heat, stir-fry rapidly but gently for 2-3 minutes. Remove fish from the skillet. Add remaining broth and stir-fry the garlic and shallot for 1 minute. Add red pepper, celery, snow peas, and water chestnuts. Cover pan and let steam for 2 minutes. In a measuring cup or small dish, combine orange juice, arrowroot, sesame oil, and vinegar. Add mixture to pan and cook until sauce thickens. Add more arrowroot, if necessary. Garnish the dish with chopped scallions. Serve over brown rice.

Most people never think to stir-fry fish! If you are gentle yet rapid, the fish should not flake and break up.

Makes 4-6 servings

STEAMED GARLIC FISH
The easiest way to prepare fish!

1 lb firm white fillets or a whole fish such as sole
1 Tbs finely chopped ginger root
2 Tbs finely minced scallions
1 Tbs tamari soy sauce
1 Tbs corn oil
1 tsp sesame oil
2 garlic cloves, peeled and sliced

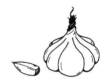

Set up a steamer or put a rack into a wok. Add about 2" of water and bring to a boil; then reduce the heat to a simmer. Put the fish on a plate large enough to accommodate it, and scatter the ginger over it. Put the plate of fish onto the steamer or rack. Cover the pan tightly and gently steam the fish until it is just cooked. Flat fish will take about 5 minutes; thicker fillets will take about 10 minutes. Remove the plate of cooked fish and sprinkle with the scallions and soy sauce. Heat the two oils together in a small saucepan. When they are hot, add the garlic slices and brown them. Pour the garlic-oil mixture over the fish. Serve immediately.

This method of preparing lean fish keeps it nice and moist. Those who usually don't like fish become converts!

Serves 4.

WHERE'S THE BEEF—*Vegetarian Meals*!

SPANISH VEGETABLE PAELLA
A great party dish!

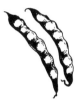

3 Tbs broth (chicken or vegetable)
1 large onion, chopped
1 clove garlic, chopped
1 medium green and red pepper, chopped
1-1/2 cups uncooked brown rice or barley
3 cups chicken broth, vegetable broth, or water
1 tsp tumeric
1 can artichoke hearts, packed in water and drained
1 cup pinto beans or black turtle beans, cooked
1 cup asparagus tips

1 tomato, cut into chunks
1 zucchini, cut into chunks
1 Tbs chopped black olives—garnish

Heat broth in a wok or heavy skillet. Saute the onion, garlic, pepper, and rice for 5 minutes. Add broth and tumeric, bring to a boil and cook over low heat for 15 minutes. Add the artichokes and beans. Cover and cook for 25-30 minutes until the rice is tender. During the last 5 minutes of cooking add the asparagus tips, tomatoes and zucchini and let the paella cook until the asparagus is tender but still crunchy and bright green. Garnish with the chopped black olives.

This mixture can be stuffed into parboiled red, green, and yellow peppers for a beautiful dish!

This is a one-pot meal that requires only a salad and perhaps some French bread.

LENTIL CHILI
A meatless chili!

1/4 cup water or broth
2 small onions, chopped
2 cloves garlic, minced
1 cup dried lentils or split peas
1-1/2 cups bulgur wheat (raw)
3 cups water or chicken broth or vegetable broth
2 cups canned tomatoes (California or plum)
    or 1-1/2 cups fresh plum tomatoes, cubed
2 Tbs chili powder (to taste) or 2 tsp cayenne pepper
1 Tbs cumin
Dash cinnamon

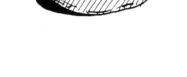

Cook the onions and garlic in water or broth in a large skillet until they are fairly tender. Add the lentils and bulgur and stir. Add water and tomatoes and stir well. Add chili powder, cumin, and cinnamon. Simmer about 30 minutes.

Variation: Add 1 can of drained kidney beans with the spices. Proceed as recipe directs.

This is great over a baked potato, brown rice, or pasta. It freezes well too. It will last 6-8 months in the freezer.

Serves 6.

PASTA FAGIOLI
This is a warm-your-insides dish!

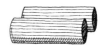

2 Tbs chicken or vegetable broth
1 large onion, chopped
3 cloves garlic, minced
2 medium carrots, sliced
2 medium zucchini, sliced
2 tsp dried basil or 1 Tbs fresh basil
2 tsp dried oregano or 1 Tbs fresh oregano
1 can (32 oz) unsalted whole tomatoes, liquid reserved (plum or California)
2 cans (16 oz each) white cannelini or navy beans, drained and rinsed for one minute

1 lb rigatoni or medium shells (whole-wheat)
Freshly ground pepper

Begin heating water to cook the pasta. Heat the broth in a large skillet on medium heat and cook the onions and garlic, stirring occasionally until softened. Add the carrots, zucchini, basil, oregano, the tomatoes with their liquid, and the beans. Cook until the vegetables are tender, about 10 minutes. Season with pepper to taste. While the vegetables are cooking, boil the pasta until tender but firm, about 7 minutes. Divide the pasta among 8 plates and spoon the vegetables and sauce on top.

This sauce may be frozen and kept for 6 months! It tastes wonderful over chicken, turkey, shrimp, or over rice!

Serves 8.

VEGETABLE LO MEIN

I have always loved lo mein served in Chinese restaurants. Even though it contains many vegetables, the fat content is too high in many restaurants. So here is my own version!

6 oz (almost 1/3 of a box) thin spaghetti
  (try whole-wheat noodles or soba noddles)
2 Tbs chicken or vegetable broth
3 scallions, minced fine
2 cloves garlic, minced fine
1 tsp fresh minced ginger
  (to mince: peel skin off the ginger,
  make two thin slices, stack on top of
  each other: slice downward into strips,
  and mince the strips)

2 medium carrots, sliced thin on the diagonal
2 medium stalks celery,
  sliced thin on the diagonal
1/2 cup sliced mushrooms (button or shiitake)
2 cups broccoli florets
1 cup vegetable or chicken broth
1 tbs arrowroot
1 tbs dry sherry
1 tbs tamari soy sauce
1 tsp sesame oil

Cook spaghetti, drain, set aside. Meanwhile, in a heavy skillet or wok, heat the broth. Add scallions, garlic, and ginger. Stir for 30 seconds. Add carrots, celery, and mushrooms and stir-fry 2 minutes more. Stir in 1/2 cup chicken broth, cover, and simmer for 3 minutes. Add broccoli, simmer 3 minutes. Meanwhile, in a small bowl or measuring cup, combine remaining chicken broth with arrowroot, soy sauce, sherry, and sesame oil. Stir until the arrowroot dissolves. Add sauce to the vegetables and cook, stirring constantly until mixture thickens, about 3 minutes. Add cooked spaghetti and toss well.

MEXICALI PIZZA
Easy as pie!

4 corn tortillas (yellow or blue)—available next to the cheeses in the refrigerated section of the market.
1 cup tomato sauce or salsa
1/2 cup low-fat cheese or crumbled tofu
Sliced jalapenos

Preheat oven to 375 degrees. Place tortillas on a baking sheet and spread with sauce, cheese or tofu, and jalapenos.

Bake for 8–10 minutes or until hot and bubbly.

Cut into triangles for a delectable appetizer. For a hearty lunch or quick dinner, just add a salad and vegetables.

Serves 4.

WHITE BEAN CHILI

1/4 cup vegetable broth or white wine
1 onion, chopped
3 garlic cloves, minced
3 Tbs minced green pepper
2 Tbs whole-wheat pastry flour or unbleached white flour
1 Tbs cumin
1-1/2 cups vegetable broth or chicken broth (if not a vegetarian)
3 cups cooked white navy beans or cannelini beans
1 cup white corn (frozen or fresh)
Minced Italian parsley for garnish

In a large stockpot, heat the broth or wine. Add onion, garlic, and green pepper. Saute for 3-4 minutes. Sprinkle flour and cumin over the onion mixture and cook one more minute. Add the remaining ingredients and bring to a boil. Lower the heat to simmer, cover, and cook for 35-45 minutes. Garnish with parsley.

Makes 6-8 servings.

INDIAN RICE CHICKPEA CURRY
My version of an easy skillet dish. Dinner in a flash!

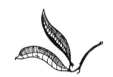

2 tsp olive oil
1/4 cup chopped onion
1/4 tart apple, chopped
1 Tbs curry powder
1 tsp garam masala (a wonderful blend of exotic Indian spices, including anise, my favorite. It can be purchased at gourmet stores as well as Indian grocers.)
3 cups cooked brown rice
2 cups cooked chick peas, drained
1/2 cup currants or raisins

Heat the oil in a skillet. Saute the onion and apple for 3 minutes to soften. Add the curry and the garam masala and cook for 1 minute. Add the rice, beans, and currants to the pan. Remove from heat and serve.

A wonderful use for leftover, cooked rice.

Serves 4.

FUSILLI WITH SAGE AND PEPPERS

With more vitamin C than citrus, a dish made with peppers is not only healthy but looks pretty too! Use the sauce over rice or a baked potato for a different topping.

1/4 cup chicken broth or vegetable broth or white wine
1 medium onion, coarsely chopped
1/2 each of red, yellow, green and orange peppers (try to find as many different peppers as you can, if you only have two or three, that is fine), cut into thin strips
3 cloves garlic, minced
1 Tbs fresh sage, minced
1 cup tomato sauce, canned or your own homemade
2 tsp tomato paste
2 Tbs dry red wine
1/8 tsp red pepper flakes (optional. Add if you want a little kick!)
fresh ground pepper
1 lb fusilli, cooked or other shaped pasta such as rigatoni or penne

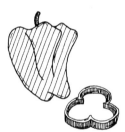

To make the sauce, in a large skillet over medium heat, heat broth or wine. Saute the onion for 2 minutes. Add the garlic, peppers and sage. Saute for 3 more minutes. Add the tomato sauce, tomato paste and red wine. Bring to a boil, lower the heat and let simmer for 10 minutes. Add the red pepper flakes and fresh pepper. Pour the sauce on each portion of cooked fusilli.

Maked 6 servings.

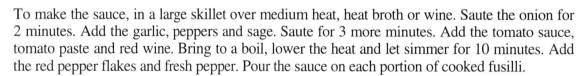

VEGETABLE BURRITOS

Here's a burrito without all the fat laden cheese! It's chock full of ingredients that are high on fiber and taste but low on the bad stuff!!!

4 whole-wheat tortillas (available at gourmet stores, some health food stores and major supermarkets. Although flour tortillas are not *the worst*, try for whole-wheat!)

2 Tbs vegetable broth
2 cloves garlic, minced
1 yellow onion, minced
1 red pepper, diced
1 cup yellow corn, cooked
    (off the cob or frozen)

1 cup cooked black beans
    (canned or from scratch), mashed slightly
1 Tbs chili powder
2 tsp cumin
1 tsp chopped cilantro
Your favorite salsa (use the one in this book!)

Wrap tortillas in foil and keep warm in a 300 degree oven or cook them, dry, in a skillet, one at a time, 1 minute on each side, and keep warm until assembly time.

To prepare the filling: Heat broth in a large skillet or wok. Add garlic, onions, and red pepper. Saute for 2 minutes. Add the corn and beans and cook another 2 minutes. Add chili powder, cumin, and cilantro. Cook an additional 1 minute.

To assemble: Spoon some bean/corn mixture on one end of each tortilla. Fold in two sides of the tortilla, roll carefully to encase the filling. Repeat. Serve with salsa.

Makes 4 tortillas.

CURRIED POTATO PUDDING
No bowls necessary, just a blender or food processor!

4 cups diced potatoes (russet or white), peeled
2 eggs (or 1 egg and 1 egg white)
1 medium onion, chopped
1/2 cup whole-wheat cracker crumbs
1 Tbs curry powder
1 tsp cumin
1/2 tsp cardamon
1/2 tsp cinnamon

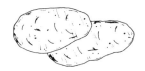

Preheat oven to 375 degrees. In a blender, combine potatoes, eggs, and onions. Stir in crumbs, curry powder, cumin, cardamon, and cinnamon.

Pour into an oiled, 2-quart baking dish or a deep 9" or 10" pie plate. Bake for 45 minutes or until firm.

Cut into squares—larger ones to serve as a side dish or smaller ones to use as an appetizer! They are great either way!

BOW TIE PASTA WITH SUN DRIED TOMATO PESTO AND WHITE BEANS

This dish not only makes one of the most filling meals but it packs an extra boost of fiber from the addition of beans. If you can't find bow ties then substitute any shaped pasta you like.

1 lb bow tie noodles, cooked al dente (just until tender, slightly chewy) and set aside

Sauce:
1 cup sun dried tomatoes, rehydrated (do not buy the sun dried tomatoes in oil)
1/4 cup non fat ricotta cheese
1 Tbs olive oil
1 Tbs pine nuts, toasted (to toast: place nuts in a dry skillet, and over medium heat shake the pan until the nuts are lightly toasted, watch carefully the nuts don't burn)
1/4 cup chopped fresh basil

2 Tbs chopped Italian parsley
1 tsp freshly grated parmesan cheese
fresh ground pepper

2 cups cooked white beans
  (cannelini or navy beans)
Italian parsley for garnish

Cook the bow tie noodles and set aside. In a blender or food processor combine all the sauce ingredients until well blended. In a saucepan combine the cooked beans and the sauce and heat until warmed throughout. To serve: on each plate, place the cooked bow ties first, top with beans mixed with pesto. Garnish with parsley.

Serves 6.

STRIVE FOR FIVE—*Eat your vegetables!*

STEWED CHAYOTE SQUASH
Chayote (shy-o-tee) is a wonderful Mexican vegetable!

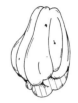

1 lb chayote squash or zucchini
2 tsp olive oil
1 medium onion, chopped
2 cloves garlic, thinly sliced
1 large tomato, chopped

Peel and pit chayote; cut into small chunks. Heat the oil over medium heat. Add onion and garlic; cook about 5 minutes, stirring often. Add the squash and tomato. Reduce the heat, cover and simmer for about 20 minutes.

Chayote is used primarily in Mexican cuisine. It is also called mirliton in Southern United States. The skin is easily removed with a vegetable peeler.

You can find chayote at Thai grocers, Health Food stores, and some major supermarkets. It tastes similar to, but better than, zucchini.

Makes 4 servings.

MUSHROOM MEDLEY
Delicious as a side dish or on top of pasta, rice, or potatoes.

10 large shiitake mushrooms (dried or fresh)
1 cup canned Chinese straw mushrooms
1/2 cup button mushrooms
1 Tbs broth
1 tsp soy sauce
2 Tbs sherry
1 tsp honey
2 tsp garlic, minced
1/3 cup chicken broth
2 Tbs finely chopped scallions

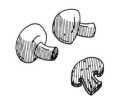

Soak shiitake mushrooms in warm water for 20 minutes, then drain, rinse well, and squeeze out any excess liquid. Discard any tough stems. Slice the caps and set aside. Drain and rinse the straw mushrooms, but leave them whole. Wipe clean the button mushrooms and slice.

Heat a wok or skillet, then add broth. Now add the mushrooms and stir-fry for a few seconds. Add soy sauce, sherry, honey, garlic, and chicken broth. Lower the heat and cook, stirring, for 7 minutes until the mushrooms are cooked. Mix in scallions. Serve.

Serves 4-6.

LEMONGRASS VEGETABLES
A nice medley of crunchy vegetables with a zip of spice!

1 Tbs corn oil
3-4 red chili peppers, chopped
1 stalk of lemongrass,
  finely chopped
1 leek, white part only, rinsed
  and thinly sliced

1 cup chicken broth
1 red pepper, sliced
1 cup fresh snow peas, trimmed
5 large shiitake mushrooms, sliced
1/2 cup canned baby corn, left whole
2 Tbs tamari soy sauce

Heat the oil in a wok or skillet. Add lemongrass, chili peppers, and leek. Stir-fry 1 minute. Add chicken broth, vegetables, and soy sauce. Cover and cook until vegetables are tender.

Goes well with brown rice for a filling vegetarian meal!

Makes 4 servings.

Note: Lemongrass, also known as citronella, is a wonderfully aromatic addition to dishes. Used extensively in Thai cuisine, lemongrass stalks can be found in some gourmet food stores and Thai grocers. To use: take the bottom portion of the stalk, about 2"-3" of it and chop into pieces. It has a delicious lemon taste.

MULTI-COLORED PEPPER STIR-FRY
Beautiful to look at!

1 Tbs chicken broth or water
2 medium-sized carrots, peeled and cut into matchstick strips
1/2 each, medium-sized sweet red pepper, yellow pepper, and green pepper cored, seeded, and cut into matchstick strips
3/4 lb snow peas or sugar snap peas, trimmed
1 Tbs tamari soy sauce
Dash black pepper

Heat the broth in a large skillet. Add carrots and red pepper and cook, covered, for 3 minutes. Add snow peas, cover, and cook 3 minutes longer or until vegetables are tender. Stir in tamari soy sauce and black pepper.

Serves 4.

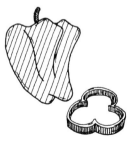

GOLDEN VEGETABLE COMBO

Kids will like this dish. It's bright color is a welcome change from green vegetables!

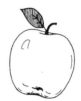

1 cup sliced golden delicious apples
2 cups thinly sliced yellow squash
1-1/2 cups thinly sliced carrots
1 small lemon, unpeeled and thinly sliced
2 tsp cinnamon
1 Tbs golden raisins
2 tsp honey
1 tsp nutmeg
1/2 cup water

Combine all ingredients in a steamer, with the water on the bottom of the pot. Cover and steam over low heat for 5 minutes until carrots are barely tender.

Serves 4.

GRILLED PORTOBELLO MUSHROOM

Portobello mushrooms are the grande dame of the mushroom world. They are very large, have a robust, meaty flavor, and are usually found at gourmet stores or at some health food stores. You can't miss them!

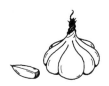

1 large portobello mushroom
1/2 Tbs olive oil
1 Tbs balsamic vinegar
1 clove garlic, minced
1 Tbs chopped fresh basil

To prepare the mushroom, cut off the stem and dust off any dirt on the cap with a paper towel or mushroom brush. In a small bowl combine the oil, vinegar, garlic, and basil. With a pastry brush, brush the cap and underneath the cap with the oil and vinegar mixture. Using either broiler or grill, place the mushroom on broiler pan or grill rack and cook for about 5-7 minutes turning once—until the mushroom is soft and has a nice grilled color. Then slice into 1/2 inch slices and eat or add slices to green salads, pastas, and pasta sauces, or over chicken.

Serves 2-4.

BROCCOLI WITH SESAME SEEDS AND SCALLIONS

Broccoli should be cooked only until its color becomes bright green. There is nothing more distasteful than limp, army-green broccoli! My favorite method is blanching, directions for which are included. You may steam your broccoli on the stovetop or in the microwave. Just make sure it comes out crunchy and beautiful to look at.

1-1/2 lbs broccoli (generally about 1 large bundle). Cut into florets. Peel the stems, if necessary, and slice into 1/2 inch pieces.
6 cups water
2 cloves garlic, minced
3 scallions, minced
2 Tbs rice vinegar
2 tsp sesame oil
1 Tbs sesame seeds

In a large pot, boil the water and then add the broccoli. Boil 1 minute, turn off the heat. Drain. Place the broccoli* into a bowl of cold water, drain again. In a large bowl, combine garlic, scallions, vinegar, sesame oil, and sesame seeds. Add broccoli and toss well. Serve at room temperature.

*Save that water in which you boiled the broccoli! Place into ice cube trays, freeze, and use whenever you need liquid as a base for soups or sauteing, instead of using oil. The water is nutrient rich from the broccoli. Just pop out the amount you need from the ice cube tray and heat.

Serves 4.

FESTIVE SWEET POTATOES

Forget the gobs of butter and brown sugar. Pineapple and spices add flavor but not unwanted calories and fat.

4 sweet potatoes
2 cups crushed pineapple, in its own juice
2 tsp cinnamon
1 tsp nutmeg
1 Tbs slivered almonds (garnish)

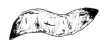

In a large saucepan, boil the unpeeled sweet potatoes over medium heat for 45 minutes or until you can pierce them easily with a fork; or bake them directly on the rack in a preheated 375 degree oven for 45 minutes to 1 hour. After completing either method of cooking, let the potatoes cool and then gently peel them. Mash the potatoes with the pineapple and spices. Place in a 1 quart casserole dish and top with slivered almonds. Bake for 20 minutes at 350 degrees.

Makes 4-6 servings.

PITA PIZZA PIZAZZ
A quick dinner! Great for lunch or dinner for the kids!

1 whole-wheat or white pita round
3 oz ground chicken, turkey, or lean beef, cooked
1 tomato, cored and thinly sliced
1/4 cup finely diced zucchini
2 Tbs your favorite tomato sauce
1/4 cup your favorite low-fat cheese, grated

Heat the broiler. Place the pita on a baking sheet and slit it completely around to form two circles. Set the top aside. Place chicken, turkey, or beef over the pita bottom, top with vegetables.

Pour sauce over the vegetables and place cheese on top. Broil until cheese melts—about 5-7 minutes. Remove the pita from the heat and cover with the pita top. Cut into wedges and serve.

The meat is optional. This treat is a vegetarian delight!

Makes 8 wedges

POTATO SKINS
Half the fat of restaurant-style potato skins!

2 large potatoes, baked
olive oil (put olive oil into a plant sprayer or cosmetic bottle to control the amount)
garlic powder
2/3 cup cheese of your choice (low-fat mozzarella)

Preheat oven to 350 degrees. Cut potatoes in half and scoop out almost all of the pulp, leaving some intact. Cut each potato half into finger size pieces. Spray some olive oil onto each piece. Sprinkle with garlic powder and top with some cheese. Bake the skins until crisp and cheese has melted.

Take the potato pulp and make mashed potatoes with skim milk, a little olive oil, and fresh herbs (1 tsp each of rosemary, thyme, or your choice).

Kids like to prepare these!

Makes at least 10 to 14 pieces.

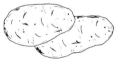

CHICKEN OF THE SEA
Great for kids of all ages!

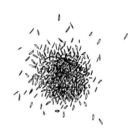

2-1/2 cups cooked chicken, cut into 1/4 inch cubes
1/2 cup seedless grapes, halved (green or red)
1/4 cup plain yogurt
2 Tbs low-fat mayonnaise
1 Tbs sesame seeds
12 jumbo pasta shells, white or whole-wheat, cooked and drained

In a serving bowl, combine chicken with the grapes, yogurt, and mayonnaise. Stuff mixture evenly into the pasta shells. Sprinkle with sesame seeds. Wrap the shells and you can take these for lunch.

Children like to prepare this dish. Grapes and chicken are a very pleasing combination. Makes 12 shells.

Serves 4-6

CAROB BROWNIES

Perfect to make on a rainy day. So easy, we don't know who will make them more, you or your kids!

1/2 cup unsweetened applesauce
1/2 cup honey or 1/4 cup honey and 1/4 cup unsweetened apple juice concentrate
1 egg and 1 egg white
1 tsp vanilla
1/3 cup carob powder or cocoa
2/3 cup whole wheat pastry flour
2 tsp baking powder
1/2 cup chopped walnuts (optional)

Preheat the oven to 325. Beat together the applesauce, honey, egg, egg white and vanilla. Combine the carob, whole wheat pastry flour and baking powder. Add to the applesauce mixture. Stir in the nuts. Pour the mixture into an oiled 8x8 baking pan. Bake for 20 to 25 minutes. Cool. Cut into squares.

Makes about 12 brownies.

OATMEAL-RAISIN COOKIES
Fun to bake anytime! A great, healthful snack for kids!

3 cups rolled oats
1 cup whole-wheat pastry flour
1 tsp baking soda
2 tsp cinnamon
1/2 cup raisins
1/4 cup applesauce
3/4 cup honey
2 eggs
1/2 cup plain nonfat yogurt
1 tsp vanilla

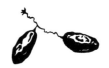

Preheat the oven to 350 degrees. Combine oats, flour, baking soda, cinnamon, and raisins. In a large bowl, beat applesauce, honey, eggs, yogurt, and vanilla until creamy. Add dry ingredients and mix well. Spray cookie sheet with no-stick spray. Drop by rounded teaspoonsful onto cookie sheet and bake 12-15 minutes.

Makes 4 dozen cookies.

FRUIT SHAKES
A nice snack or quick breakfast. The blender does the work, you get the taste!

Basic Mix:
1 cup skim milk
1 cup fresh fruit
1 tsp vanilla
2 tsp honey
3-4 large ice cubes

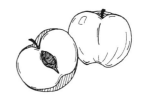

Place all ingredients into a blender and blend until smooth.

Fruit Options:
1 banana, peeled
1 cup strawberries, stemmed and washed
1 cup cut up peaches
1 cup blueberries

Makes 2 servings.

138 **SWEET ENDINGS**—*Delicious desserts!*

STRAWBERRIES WITH STRAWBERRY SAUCE
Refreshing, easy, and light!

2 pints fresh strawberries
2 tsp honey
2 Tbs orange juice
Fresh blueberries for garnish

For each serving, leave the strawberries whole and divide the pint among the dessert dishes. To make sauce, puree the remaining pint of strawberries with the honey and orange juice. Strain to remove any seeds. Pour a little sauce over each dish and top with a few fresh blueberries.

Place in fluted champagne glasses for an unusually spectacular dessert!

Serves 6.

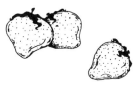

PAPAYA MOUSSE

Select papayas with smooth skin that give a little!

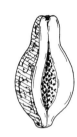

2 papayas, peeled, seeded, chopped into small chunks
1/2 cup plain yogurt or part skim ricotta cheese
1 banana, peeled
1 tsp vanilla or almond extract
1-2 tsp honey
3-4 large ice cubes
Kiwi slices or strawberries

Place all ingredients in a blender and blend until very smooth. Refrigerate overnight to thicken. Place in dessert dishes and top with a kiwi slice or a strawberry.

If you use a crystal bowl and decorate with the kiwis and strawberries, you will have a most elegant dessert!

(You can use peaches or strawberries instead of the papaya.)

Serves 4.

HOT FRUIT COMPOTE
So nice on a cold winter day!

3 cups mixed canned fruit in their own juice
1/2 cup dried apricots
1 cup raisins
1/2 tsp cinnamon
1/4 tsp ground nutmeg
1/2 cup brandy
2 Tbs fresh lemon juice
2 Tbs honey

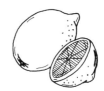

Preheat oven to 350 degrees. Layer the fruit in a casserole dish. Scatter raisins over the fruit. Sprinkle with cinnamon and nutmeg. Place the brandy and lemon juice in a bowl. Stir in honey. Pour over the fruit. Bake for 30 minutes or until heated through.

This dish is good for people who require their fruits to be cooked for easier digestion.

BROWN RICE PUDDING
Comforting and good! Have for breakfast—why not?

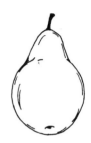

3 eggs (or 1 egg and 2 egg whites)
1-1/2 cups skim milk
1/2 cup honey
1 tsp vanilla
1 tsp lemon peel
2 tsp lemon juice
1/2 tsp cinnamon
1/2 tsp nutmeg
2 apples or pears, cored and chopped (Granny Smith apples or D'Anjou pears are lovely!)
1/2 cup raisins or currants (optional)
2 cups brown rice, cooked

Preheat the oven to 325 degrees. Beat together the eggs, milk, and honey. Stir in vanilla, lemon peel, lemon juice, spices, apples, and rice. Pour mixture into a buttered baking dish and bake for 50 minutes, until set.

Grain, low-fat dairy, and fruit—all in one tasty dish!

Serve warm or cold.

BLUEBERRY BAKE
Something like Grandma's, this dessert is sweet and delicious!

Filling:

1/4 cup honey

1 Tbs arrowroot

1/2 tsp cinnamon

4 cups blueberries or blackberries (fresh or frozen)

1 cup water

2 Tbs lemon juice

Crust:

1 cup whole-wheat pastry flour

1 tsp baking powder

1 Tbs honey

1/2 tsp baking soda

1/2 cup buttermilk

Preheat oven to 400 degrees. Thoroughly combine honey, arrowroot, and cinnamon in a medium saucepan. Stir in lemon juice, fruit, and water. Bring the mixture to a boil over medium heat. Stir gently. Simmer for 3-4 minutes and then pour into a 1-1/2 quart casserole dish.

Combine flour, baking powder, and baking soda in a large bowl. Add honey and buttermilk. Stir to blend. Drop tablespoons of dough on the hot fruit, completely covering it, or make a pattern. Can be made with any fruit. Bake for 20 minutes.

Makes 8 servings.

BREAD PUDDING WITH LEMON SAUCE
Try it with whole-wheat raisin bread!

5 to 6 cups diced whole-wheat bread
1 cup diced apple or pear or peach
1 egg and 3 egg whites
4 cups skim milk
1/3 cup honey
2 tsp vanilla extract
1 tsp cinnamon
Lemon sauce (see next recipe)

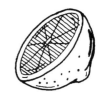

Mix bread and apples in a greased 9" x 13" or 2-quart baking dish. Beat eggs and egg whites with milk, honey, and vanilla. Pour over bread and let stand for 15 minutes to soften and absorb the liquid. Preheat the oven to 350 degrees. Sprinkle surface of pudding with cinnamon. Bake for about 30-40 minutes until custard is set and lightly browned.

Serves 10.

LEMON SAUCE
Wonderful topping—as tart as you like it!

1 Tbs arrowroot
1/4 cup honey
1 tsp grated lemon rind
1 cup water
1/4 cup lemon juice

Mix arrowroot, honey, lemon rind, and water in a small saucepan. Bring to boiling over medium heat. Boil, stirring constantly, for 5 minutes. Remove from heat and blend in lemon juice. If sauce is too tart, add a bit more honey. Serve over bread pudding.

BLUEBERRY GINGERBREAD

*Jeanette's done it again! Here is her recipe for gingerbread adding blueberries.
DDDDD..Delicious!!*

1 1/2 cups unbleached all purpose flour
1 cup whole wheat pastry flour
1 tsp baking soda
1 tsp baking powder
1 tsp cinnamon
2 tsp ground ginger
1/4 cup honey

1/3 cup blackstrap molasses
2 Tbs canola oil or 2 Tbs
    unsweetened applesauce
1/2 cup nonfat buttermilk
1 large egg
2 large egg whites
1 cup fresh or frozen blueberries

Prehaet oven to 350 degrees. Coat and 8 x 8 inch baking pan with cooking spray or lightly oil.

Sift the flours and spices together into a large bowl and set aside.

Combine buttermilk, honey, molasses, and canola oil, mix well. Add egg and egg whites and beat well. Combine the buttermilk mixture and blueberries with the flour mixture. Stir by hand until just combined.

Pour into prepared pan. Bake for 45 minutes or until tootpick inserted in center comes out clean. Cool cake on wire rack. Dust cake with confectioners sugar, if desired. Cut into squares and serve.

APPLE CRANBERRY CRISP
Can be eaten for breakfast!

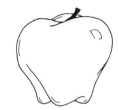

7 apples (Granny Smiths are great!), cored and sliced
1 cup cranberries, whole or chopped
2 Tbs lemon juice
1 tsp cinnamon
1 tsp nutmeg
1/4 cup whole-wheat pastry flour
1/2 cup rolled oats
2 Tbs sunflower oil (more, if needed) or canola oil
2 Tbs honey (more, if needed)
1 tsp vanilla

Lay all the apple slices and cranberries into an 8" x 8" baking dish. Combine lemon juice and spices in a small bowl; pour over apple slices and cranberries. Combine flour, oats, oil, honey, and vanilla. Mix until mixture resembles granola. Sprinkle over apples and cranberries and bake at 325 degrees for 20 minutes. Broil 2 minutes, until top is slightly browned, if desired.
(Omit the cranberries if you just like, and just have apple crisp)
You can also substitute peaches or pears!

Serves 6-8.

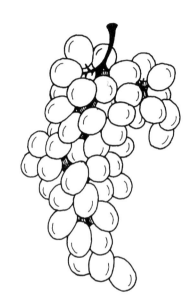

APPENDIX I

Pinch of Thyme Cooking School

Robyn Webb's A Pinch of Thyme Cooking School will give you the recipe for a whole new world of delicious and nutritious cooking possibilities. And you'll learn to prepare, in minutes, interesting meals that everyone will love.

Just imagine preparing gourmet delights like Turkey Provincal, Pasta Fagioli, or Mango Mousse—and not feeling guilty! You don't have to, because at Robyn Webb's A Pinch of Thyme Cooking School you can learn to prepare fabulous meals without sugar and with minimal amounts of fat and sodium.

Robyn Webb helps you take the mystery out of low-fat cooking by teaching you how to alter your old recipes and create a delicious low-fat alternative. You'll add excitement to your cooking possibilities once you've learned Robyn Webb's recipe to...Save Time, Add Flavor, and Lower Fat!

Promises of the Courses:

- You will have a new sense of ease and confidence when preparing meals.

- You will know how to enhance the flavors and appearance of foods without adding extra fat.

- You will learn new cooking techniques that are easy and quick to prepare. You will know how to stock your kitchen and what products to buy.

- Cooking will become fun and exciting.

A *Pinch of Thyme* on the move: If you can't come to us we'll come to you! Our cooking school can come to your location and teach any course listed in this brochure or customize a course for YOU. You provide the space, we take care of the rest! A perfect idea for a wedding or baby shower, birthday party or simply getting friends together for an educational, fun time. Minimum of 15 participants required. Inquire about pricing.

COURSE DESCRIPTIONS

Basic Curriculum: The following three courses have been designed to give you all the special skills you need to cook low-fat, time-saving meals with flavor! You may take the courses in any order desired. Each course is two sessions. A full dinner and complete recipe and information packet are provided at each session.

We've Only Just Begun
An Introduction to Nutritional Cooking This practical *how-to* course is a must for everyone from the kitchen phobic to the gourmet who wants to cook in a more healthful way. We strongly suggest you participate in this course first.

Session 1
Another Piece of Chicken? Poultry is often prescribed for a low-fat diet, but all too often it becomes tiresome. In this first session you will discover the techniques to prepare chicken in various ways that are simple and fast, but never boring! All the recipes are appropriate for everyday or for company. Includes instruction on how to buy and store chicken.

Session 2
The Daily Catch—Delicious Fish: Now you don't have to wait to eat fish at a restaurant. We'll expose the *secrets* in cooking fish, so its perfect every time. Learn to prepare *the catch of the day*, utilizing poaching, sauteing, broiling and marinating techniques that seal in flavor. Included are instructions on how to store, prepare, and cook fabulous fish.

Where's the Beef?
Vegetarian cuisine 1990's Style: Whether you want to go to meatless once a week or become a vegetarian, you will find this cuisine is versatile and can appeal to everyone.

Session 1
Cooking with Beans and Grains: We'll introduce you to the exciting world of many different grains and beans. No longer relegated as side dishes, you will learn how to prepare main meals so good that no one will ask, *Where's the meat?* Since vegetarian cooking is so versatile, all the recipes can become new recipes by simply varying the beans, grains, or spices. Included will be how to purchase, store and cook all types of grains and beans.

Session 2
Not Taboo Any More—Pizza and Pasta: Yes, you can indulge in long time favorites, pasta and pizza—Robyn's way. Learn to prepare more than just spaghetti and tomato sauce and enjoy pizza without the guilt. Many types and shapes of pasta will be used and various pizza crusts will be prepared. Includes discussion on how to purchase, store, and cook pasta.

Around The World
Healthy Foods from Different Lands: Around the World is designed to get your creative juices flowing! You will learn to make ethnic foods nutritious, without eliminating authenticity. The recipes are easy and innovative.

Session 1
Italian—Mediterranean Made Healthy: Learn to prepare appetizers, salads, vegetables, main courses and desserts that are brimming with robust flavors and textures, highlighting the Tuscany region of Italy. Discussion on where to purchase special ingredients. Explore how to choose the best dishes from an Italian restaurant menu, keeping health in mind.

Session 2
Chinese and Thai—East Meets West: Once the preparation is complete, Chinese and Thai cooking are the fastest food around! In this session you will learn the techniques of

stir frying, steaming, poaching, simmering and more! Create mouth watering recipes for soups, salads, vegetables, main dishes, and dessert. Instruction on proper cutting techniques and what equipment is needed will be discussed. Includes information on where to buy ingredients as well as how to select from Chinese and Thai menus.

Single Session Courses
A complete dinner (except for bread baking) and recipe packet is provided at each class.

Cooking for Singles
Time saving Meals For One Or Two: Whether you're dining alone or with a friend, this course enables you to prepare simple, nutritious and interesting meals. Learn to take shortcuts when preparing a variety of salads, vegetables, main courses with minimal cleanup and waste. We'll also show you how to get the best use of your freezer and make-ahead dishes. Having-fun-in-the-kitchen-with-delicious-results is the theme for this course.

Party Food Without Guilt
Hors D'oeuvres: Those innocent looking little finger foods are just waiting to cast disaster upon your diet at the next party! But wait, you don't have to stay home or not entertain yourself. In our calorie-saving party course, you will discover the many pleasures of preparing dips, pates, tarts and other finger foods that will please any crowd. These recipes are also suitable for people who like to **graze** for a meal. Start planning your next get together guilt free!

The Staff of Life

Bread Baking: There is nothing like a loaf of warm, crusty bread straight from the oven. Now you can learn the secrets of bakers to produce delicious aromatic bread. Join us for this very special class, when a representative from the famed Marvelous Market will teach the steps to successful baking. Class participation is limited.

Special Chefs' Night

A Pinch of Thyme is proud to present classes featuring the Washington area's outstanding and well-known chefs who share our philosophy of good food and good health. the evening program will highlight the chefs' specialties, adding up to a very satisfying meal. All the recipes will be given, so you can create these easy, delicious dishes at home. For this semester's class, please refer to the course schedule included with the brochure. Don't miss this very special night!

Thyme to Dine Out—

Dining Out At Famous Washington Restaurants: Ever wish you can go to a restaurant and not worry about ordering slathers of cream sauce on your pasta? Come and experience the talents of top Washington area chefs as we present restaurants where you will be served low-fat fare created just for A Pinch Of Thyme guests. For this semester's restaurant refer to the course date insert. Price includes full dinner, tax and gratuity.

Cooking With Five Ingredients Or Less!

One, two, three, four, five—that's all it takes to create a great meal! In this new course we will show you the fastest recipes ever created by Robyn Webb. Recipes for appetizers, salads, main courses, vegetables and dessert will be on the table in minutes. You'll save clean up as well. We'll teach you to use the staple products that you have on hand, which can be transformed into hundreds of dishes, keeping the fat low of course!

Thyme For A Season—

Seasonal Foods With A Flair: There is a season for everything! NOW, we have created this course to celebrate the change of seasons. Each semester, we will highlight the best foods of the season. We will also include seasonal food shopping tips to insure good produce buying. For this semester's class refer to the course date insert.

NUTRITIONAL COUNSELING

Private counseling is available for those who are serious about transforming the quality of their health and body image. This is not a "diet" approach to health, rather we will design a comprehensive food management program specific to your life style and unique metabolic requirements. We will provide you with all the information and support you need to become nutritionally savvy and motivated to reach and sustain your goals. For a private appointment, please call our offices.

We design programs for:

- **Weight Loss**

- **Weight Gain**

- **Cholesterol Management**

- **Fatigue**

- **Pregnancy**

A "PINCH OF THYME" CATERING

After several years of teaching low-fat, high-flavor cooking in the Washington area, we noticed *that people loved our food*. Although made with healthful ingredients, dishes like Chicken Enchiladas with Grape Salsa, Spicy Black Bean Salad, and Lemon Laced Cheesecake disappeared from people's plates!

We offer all manner of catering from buffet parties, to luncheons, to healthy corporate breakfasts. Those days of serving mundane fare at parties are over at last! For inspiring menus and to arrange a private appointment, please call our offices.

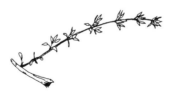

LECTURES AND SEMINARS

Now, more than ever, people require the correct information about nutrition. Robyn Webb Associates provide diverse lectures and seminars that are appropriate for the workplace, organizations, religious groups, or schools.

Topics include:

- **Decreasing Your Cravings**

- **Life in the Fat Lane**

- **Cholesterol: Get the Facts**

- **Cooking Extravaganza • Nutrition: A Family Affair • Keeping your Commitment to your Health**

Fees are charged on an hourly basis.

ROBYN WEBB ASSOCIATES (703)683-5034

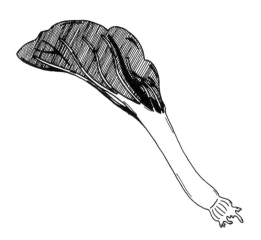

Brand Names and Shopping Resources

Here is a listing of my favorite brands of food from the Light Larder List. I am also including places to shop.

Tamari Soy Sauce: San J Lite, Ewehon, Eden

Vinegars: Rice-Eden (brown rice vinegar)

Ty Ling (white rice vinegar)

China Bowl (white rice vinegar)

Mustards: Grey Poupon (all varieties); Westbrae

Cottage Cheese: Any that is 1% milkfat or less

Part -Skim Ricotta Cheese: Polly-O Reduced Calorie Lite, Non-Fat Maggio

Whole Grain Breads: Recommended bakeries in the Metropolitian area:

Marvelous Market—Locations in Virginia and the District

Uptown Bakers—In the District

Great Harvest—In Vienna, Herndon, and Alexandria, Virginia

Springswood Bakers—Bethesda, Maryland

Bakers Place—McLean, Virginia; Chevy Chase, Maryland; Silver Spring, Maryland; and Potomac, Maryland

Firehook Bakery—Old Town Alexandria, Virginia

Fresh Fields Stores (Bread Department)—Annandale, Tysons Corner, Fairfax Station, Springfield, and Charlottesville, in Virginia; Bethesda and Rockville, in Maryland

Sutton Place Gourmet (Bread Department)—Locations in the District, Maryland, and Virginia

Giant Gourmets (Bread Department)—District, Virginia, and Maryland

Learn to make your own! Live in the area? Take my breadmaking class.

Fruits and vegetables: In addition to the fruits and vegetables you use, I have included a few exotic ones in the recipes.

Shiitake Mushrooms: Used primarily in Oriental cooking, shiitakes have a nice meaty texture and wonderful taste. You can purchase fresh ones at gourmet grocers, health food stores, and some major supermarkets. You can purchase dried ones, year round, at Oriental grocers, gourmet stores, some health food stores, and some major supermarkets. Just trim off the stem, slice, and saute.

Jicama: This Mexican potato is ugly, but delicious! You can't miss it in the store. It is brown skinned; you can peel it; then cut into slices. Serve raw for a nice, added crunch to salads. It tastes slightly sweet and has texture like a water chestnut.

Lemongrass: Also known as citronella, lemongrass will give an aromatic lemon flavor to your food. Used extensively in Thai cuisine you may use it to flavor soups, poultry, and vegetables. It looks like a stalk about 7 inches in length with a light greenish yellow color. To use, cut about 2-3 inches off the base. Use the top to flavor soups. Then peel away 2-3 layers of the outer leaves and chop the lemongrass as you would a scallion. Saute the pieces with garlic, shallots, ginger, or whatever seasoning vegetables are called for in a recipe. Then proceed with the rest of the recipe. You can find lemongrass at gourmet food shops, health food stores, Oriental grocers, and some major supermarkets.

Low Sodium Chicken Broth: Although there is a recipe for chicken broth in this book, if you don't wish to use it, you can purchase it canned. My favorite brand is the fat-free Health Valley broth. You can find Health Valley at most health food stores, gourmet stores, and some major supermarkets.

Low Sodium Canned Tomatoes: Eden

Salsa: Enricos, Hot Cha Cha, or from your favorite deli or use the recipe in this book

Dry white Wine: Chablis, Chenin Blanc, Sauvignon Blanc or Johannisberg Riesling

Dry Sherry: Taylor or Gallo for inexpensive brands; buy more expensive brands if you like.

Olive Oil: Colavita, Eden, Alessi, Santini

Sesame Oil: Kame, China Bowl, Eden

Vanilla Extract: Wagners, Old Spicery Shoppe

No Sugar Jams: Polaner All Fruit, Sorrell Ridge, McCutcheons (a local company in Frederick, Maryland that makes the best jam)

Whole-Wheat Pastry Flour: Arrowhead Mills or buy in bulk at your favorite health food store

Oats: Quaker, McCann's Irish Oatmeal, Old Wessex Irish Oatmeal

Arrowroot: Just buy in bulk at a gourmet store or health food store

Whole Wheat Pasta: If you can get fresh at a gourmet store, get it. If not, here are a few brands I'd recommend: Eden, Westbrae, DeCecco.

Buckwheat Noodles: (Also known as soba noodles) Eden or any brand at any Oriental grocer

Brown and Wild Rice: Brown Rice—Lundberg, Wild Rice—Grey Owl, available at health food stores

Bulgur Wheat: Old World or buy in bulk from a health food store or Middle Eastern store

Barley: Most brands I found acceptable, or buy from bulk section in a health food store

Lentils: Buy in bulk

Herbal Teas: There are so many companies now, but I still like Celestial Seasons because of the many interesting flavors.

Sparkling Waters and Spring Waters: Quibell, Perrier, Appolinaris are my favorites. In spring waters, my favorite is the Volvic brand, particularly the orange flavor.

You can, of course, stick with brand names you love and trust. This list will help those who may need additional assistance in finding good brands.

Stores

For many of the ingredients in this book, you can shop at just a local major supermarket. To broaden your horizons however, I am going to include a few stores that are worth the trip. If you find you can only get to these places occasionally, just stock up!

Fresh Fields Supermarkets—A good for you (as they say) store that stocks every major health food brand of canned and boxed goods, full bakery, deli, fish market, cheese and fresh pasta, floral department, vitamins and cosmetics, household cleaning supplies (environmentally friendly), and the highlight—a huge selection of the most gorgeous produce with many of the items being organic

Virginia Locations: Annandale, Charlottesville, Springfield, Tysons Corner, Fairfax Station

Maryland Locations: Annapolis, Bethesda, Rockville

There are also Fresh Fields in Philadelphia, PA and two locations in the Chicago, IL area.

Cash Grocer—1315 King Street, Old Town Alexandria

A true gem of a place with a huge selection of bulk food items—This store stocks many canned and boxed health food brands, organic produce, vitamins and cosmetics, books, herbs, breads and more.

Straight From The Crate—Richmond Highway, Alexandria, VA

Another fine store with selections of produce, boxed and canned items, and more

Healthways—Locations in: Annandale, Arlington, Fairfax Springfield, Sterling, and Manassas

An excellent store with many offerings for the health minded

Yes!—Cleveland Park, in the District

A great store with an extensive selection of canned and boxed items, books, vitamins, refrigerated products, and cosmetics

Mother Goodness—In McLean, Virginia

A handsome store with beautiful, finished-wooden tables at which to sit while dining on delicious sandwiches, salads, hot entrees, desserts, and beverages, all made to order—included are selections of canned and boxed items, vitamins, books, and more

Sutton Place Gourmet—Locations in Virginia, Maryland, and the District

Voted Best Gourmet Store, this is the epitome of gourmet food shopping. Everything imaginable for the cook and the diner—full bakery, meat department, cheeses, traiteur (take home items), wines and beers, beautiful produce, deli, coffees.

Giant Gourmets and Someplace Special—Location in McLean, Virginia. Other locations of Giant Gourmets are all over the Washington area. They have nice selections of gourmet and health food items.

For a great guide to ethnic stores, purchase the Washington Ethnic Food Store Guide, by Jim Lawson, Admore Publications, P.O. Box 21051, Washington, DC 20009. It is the best guide and I use it!

Call ahead to all stores for hours and specific locations.

Using Your Freezer

The freezer can be a great help in do-ahead preparations. But while some foods freeze well and with minimal preparation, others require special handling, and some should not be frozen at all.

DO NOT FREEZE:

Cooked egg whites and soft meringues

Gelatin

Cake or pie with custard filling

Mayonnaise

Cloves and imitation vanilla

Milk, light cream, or sour cream

Heavy cream, except when whipped

Vegetables, with high water content (celery, tomatoes,

leafy salad greens, fennel, etc., unless they have been cooked and finely chopped)

FREEZING TIPS

- Before freezing fish, dip it in lemon juice to help preserve its original taste and texture. Then wrap it snugly in plastic wrap, followed by layers of aluminum foil.

- A convenient way to freeze egg whites is in an ice cube tray one per cube. When solid, transfer the frozen egg white cubes to freezer bags.

- Fruits that freeze well include berries, citrus, figs, peaches, and cherries.

- In its frozen state, ginger is easier to peel and grate. It keeps for several months.

- When you add items to your freezer, limit them to about two pounds for each cubic foot of freezer space.

- Rotate items in the freezer so that older items aren't forgotten. Keep a list of freezer foods; when you remove an item, check it off.

Refrigerator And Freezer Storage Times

FOOD	REFRIGERATOR FREEZER	34.–40.f	or Lower
Butter:		2– weeks	6–8 months
Eggs: Hard cooked		1 week	(Do not freeze)
Whites (raw)		1 week	12 months
Yolks (raw)		2 days	6 months
Fish: Lean fish (cod, flounder)		1 day	6 months
Fat fish (salmon, bluefish)		1 day	3 months
Chicken, Turkey:		1–4 days	6–7 months
Bread: Quick (baked)		3–7 days	3 months
Yeast (baked)		7–14 days	3 months
Yeast dough		3–5 days	1 month

Fruit:

Apricots, berries, cherries	3 days	8–12 months
Melons, nectarines, peaches,	3–5 days	8–12 months
Plums, pears apples, citrus fruits, cranberries	1–2 weeks	8–12 months

Vegetables:

Corn	1 day	8–12 months
Asparagus, green beans	2–3 days	8–12 months
Artichokes, broccoli,	3–5 days	8–12 months
Collards, lima beans, peas, spinach, turnip greens,		
Winter Squash, beets, cauliflower, carrots,	2–3 weeks	8–12 months

Time Savers For the Kitchen

- The main advantage to preparing meals ahead is that you can cook when it is convenient for you. But there are extra benefits too. The following is a list of ideas to make your life easier so you have more time to spend with your family.

- By grouping tasks, you can save time overall and have fewer cleanup chores. For instance, if you double a casserole recipe and freeze half, you will spend nearly 50% less time than you would in preparing it twice. And you clean up the kitchen only once!

- Planned leftovers are another way to get more (mileage) from your cooking time. Make extra quantities of poultry, rice, and potatoes to be used in salads, soups, and more.

- When chopping onions, peppers, or garlic, triple the quantity for later use. These will keep, covered in the refrigerator, for up to one week; in the freezer for up to six months. Combined with some olive oil, minced garlic will keep for several months in the refrigerator.

- If you wash greens and herbs as soon as you get them home, they are ready whenever you need them. Spin them dry thoroughly, then store in plastic bags lined with paper towels. Depending on the type and freshness, greens will keep in the refrigerator from three to six days; herbs such as parsley and dill, will last for up to two weeks.

Grain Cookery

There are many ways to cook grains. The two most common ways are to either add grain to a boiling liquid or add a liquid to a grain. If you have trouble cooking grains, you may want to invest in a rice cooker. Some of my students swear by the cooker. Who doesn't sometimes forget there is something on the stove until it is too late! So a rice cooker will help since it shuts off when the rice or grain is cooked and you can continue to chat on the phone!

Boiling water: Sprinkle the grain slowly into double the amount of water or broth, cover the pot with a tight fitting lid, lower the heat and cook until the water is absorbed. Avoid the tendency to play chef here and try not to continuously stir while the grain cooks. When you do this, the grain will come out like a mushy mess!! Always set your kitchen timer ahead 10 minutes prior to the cooking time. You can always cook it longer

Sauteing the grain: To do this method, add 1 Tbs oil to the saucepan and saute your grain for about 5 minutes. This will bring out the tasty flavor most grains have and it is delicious. Add double the amount of water or broth, lower the heat, cover the pot with a tight fitting lid and cook until the water is absorbed.

Brown Rice	50 minutes
Kasha	20 minutes
Millet	30 minutes

Barley	60 minutes
Oats	10 minutes
Quinoa	15 minutes

For couscous and bulgur wheat you do not need a saucepan. Just add double the amount of liquid and let the liquid absorb. For couscous the water should absorb in 5 minutes and for bulgur wheat it should be 30-45 minutes or up to an hour.

Basic Bean Cookery

You may use canned beans if you want to or you can prepare them yourself. You are not personally involved in the process so although they take time to soak and cook you can be doing other things!

For people who have digestive problems with beans here are two tricks to use. There is a digestive aid on the market called BEANO. It works by putting a drop or two into the food and it does really work! You may also drop a piece of seaweed such as kombu (available at health food stores or Oriental markets) into cooking liquid.

There are two ways to soak beans, a long way and a short way. Use the regular soaking method when you have time on your hands to soak beans. Use the quick soak method when you want beans in a hurry.

Regular soak: Rinse beans in cool water. Drain. Place in a large pot with two to three times their volume of water and let stand for about eight hours.

Quick soak: Place the rinsed, drained beans in a pot with two to three times their volume of water. Bring to a boil, simmer for two minutes, cover, remove from heat, and let stand for one to two hours.

Cooking: Cooking is the same after either method: drain the beans. Bring the pot of beans and the fresh water to a boil, cover, and simmer, keeping heat low until tender. Use the timetable below to determine cooking times.

Black beans	1-1/2–2 hours
Black-eyed peas	1-1/2–2 hours
Chickpeas	1-1/2–2 hours
Kidney beans	1-1/2–2 hours
Lentils (you do not need to soak first)	45 minutes
Lima beans	45 minutes
Navy and pea beans	1-1/2–2 hours
Pinto beans	1-1/2–2 hours
Split peas (you do not need to soak first)	45 minutes
White beans	1-1/2–2 hours

Storage

BEANS

Dried: Store at room temperature in an airtight container. Will keep for more than one year. **Cooked**: In the refrigerator, will last covered for 1 week. In the **freezer** beans will last in an airtight package for 6-9 months.

GRAINS

Whole grains: Best stored at below 68. In an airtight container, will last 6-9 months. **Cooked grains:** In the refrigerator, covered, will keep for 1 week.

FLOURS

In a **cool** spot, in an airtight container, for 2-3 months In the **refrigerator**, in an airtight container, for 6 months. In the **freezer**, in an **airtight** container, for 1 year.

PASTA

Dried pasta will keep at room temperature in an airtight package for more than one year. **Fresh pasta in the refrigerator**, covered, for 1-2 days. **Fresh pasta in the freezer**, in an airtight package for 6 months. **Cooked pasta in the refrigerator**, covered, for 1 week. **Cooked pasta in the freezer** is NOT recommended.

Index

Bibliography

Nikki and David Goldbeck's American Whole Foods Cuisine by Nikki and David Goldbeck, New York, New York, Penguin Group, 1983 (for grain and bean cookery information)

The Complete Vegetarian Cuisine by Rose Elliot, New York, New York, Pantheon Books, 1988

Awaken the Giant Within by Anthony Robbins, New York, New York, 1991

Jane Brody's Good Food Book by Jane Brody, Bantam Books, 1985

Make it Easy Make it Light by Laurie B. Grad, New York, New York, Simon and Shuster, 1991

Make it Now, Cook it Later, Reader's Digest, 1989 (for freezer information)

)